STRESS LESS

*An easy and proven way
to cope & reduce stress*

DR. ZACH FAYENA

Producer & International Distributor
eBookPro Publishing
www.ebook-pro.com

Stress Less
Dr. Zach Fayena

Copyright © 2020 Zach Fayena

All rights reserved; No parts of this book may be reproduced or transmitted in any form or by any means, electronic or mechanical, including photocopying, recording, taping, or by any information retrieval system, without the permission, in writing, of the author.

Translation from the Hebrew by Jerry Hyman

Contact: zfayena@gmail.com

ISBN 9798664968774

Dedicated to my family

STRESS LESS

*An easy and proven way
to cope & reduce stress*

DR. ZACH FAYENA

Contents

INTRODUCTION

Often, when asked if I am engaged in a high-pressure occupation, I pause for a moment, searching for the right response and usually answer, "Yes. Fortunately, my occupation is stressful." The answer may seem odd, as most of us associate stress with a threat or something negative. If that is so, why do I choose to say "yes"?

Before answering this question, here is an illustration of what I mean by my answer. Each of us, no matter what our occupation (garage owner, physician, staff manager, or teacher) identify with the role we play in society and its significance in our lives. We most likely have two simultaneous sensations: on the one hand, a feeling of "keeping to ourselves," and on the other, heavy responsibility.

We keep to ourselves because we think that if we share our feelings with others around us, our self-image will be damaged, since the identity we have created for ourselves – with the support of those around us – is that we are strong, we are leaders, people who do not break down, but always move forward…and other such clichés.

"Keeping to ourselves," manifests itself in thoughts such as, "who can I share my feelings with when I am hurting or having a hard time?" It is interesting to note that even people who are surrounded by love and human affection can still feel lonely when they are faced with a stressful situation.

It doesn't matter if we are managers, workers, business owners, or whether we have a family or are single, we all must take responsibility, and many of us will describe it as a heavy responsibility. We tend to describe this feeling of taking responsibility with expressions such as: "a heavy load," "the burden of proof is on me," "it's a weight on my shoulders," "other people's expectations from me," and more.

From this perspective, responsibility has mostly a negative meaning. Examples of such responsibility are many and varied.

For example, let's take the CEO of a large, successful company. Such a person has a professional responsibility to the employees, managers, shareholders, and customers of the company. On a personal level, he bears responsibility for his children, his parents, his friends, and others around him.

The question arises: Who are we fooling? Who are we lying to? We have already pointed out that whatever your occupation, the symptoms will be the same. This bridge between the image we create for ourselves and what actually happens, can lead many of us to feel exhaustion, and sometimes can even lead to a breakdown – a feeling that everything is closing in on us and we cannot breathe.

The bravest of us will admit it and try to address these feelings, but most of us will simply push the feelings away and convince ourselves that this is just how it is. We say to ourselves that we need to make a living, we need to take care of the family, and so on. Even if we are not happy with what we are doing, we tell ourselves we don't know anything else we can do. We will continue to blame others and think the problem is around us and not within us. Some will suffer from physical symptoms, others from mental symptoms, but must of us will suffer from both.

However, stress can be a positive factor in our lives. It pushes us to engage in social activity, and also makes us seek meaning and purpose in our lives. Not long ago, a friend consulted me on whether he ought to choose an intense and busy role with lots of pressure, or one that he thinks will be calmer and less stressful.

For me, the answer is quite simple, and it is backed by scientific findings. It is always better to choose a job or occupation that is significant for you. It is better to live a meaningful life and learn to regulate stress, rather than choose a job or workplace where the subjective stress index is low. By the way, I can promise you that everywhere, and in every situation there will always be factors that you have to deal with that can put you under stress in one way or another.

In any case, to deal with stress it is advisable to learn techniques that will enable you to regulate stress so that its negative effect is low and its positive effect high. In addition, I offer you a slightly different approach. I suggest to you to avoid all kinds of recommendations for how to live a balanced life, etc. After all, what is balance? Everyone has their own individual balance point. The desire for balance that is almost impossible to achieve, causes a feeling of stress of its own.

By the way, did you know that stress makes us more social beings? Science has found that the hormone oxytocin (commonly known as the "love hormone") or in its masculine version, vasopressin, is secreted in part by expressing social empathy and causing us at a certain point to want to hug someone who needs a hug, or allows a mother after giving birth, to bond with her newborn infant. The secreted hormone can also enable us to recognize when friends are in stressful situations, and to be empathetic toward them and thus, be social beings who can help others.

In this book, I will try to share with you the insights that I have accumulated during my life to regulate stress – precisely that: "regulate stress." I have deliberately avoided terms such "stress-free living," a "balanced life," "overcoming stress," and so on. I prefer to use terms like "regulating stress" or "coping with stress," as they imply a sense of control over how we choose to live our lives.

This book is a product of my life's journey, and in my humble opinion, many will see in it analogies to their life's journey as well, as we all cope with stress. The difference is in how we choose to do it, or in other words, how we choose to live our lives.

On my life's journey, I have chosen to perceive several points in my life from a different perspective and also to give you, my readers, a fresh slant on familiar situations. Seeing things from a new perspective allows a different interpretation of what happens to us in life. By dealing with the difficulties, we actually go through a process of self-observation.

I learned this about myself: that even in times of enormous struggle and moments when you feel an abyss opening up underneath you, even then, you will discover that every crisis has meaning.

I have learned that a crisis does not only mean the end of

something, but also a starting point. The crisis has meaning and if we listen for it, even from the depths of gloom, we can find hope.

I have allowed myself to write this book not from the point of view of a psychologist, a doctor, or therapist, as I do not practice any of these important professions. Instead, I have written this book out of personal curiosity, life experience, and academic knowledge. The skills at my command have led me to ask the right questions, to look for the most reliable and valid answers, and to provide a simple, practical, and structured perspective on coping with stress for myself and for my readers

In the coming chapters, I will describe to you my personal journey in attempting to decipher the stress response. The book is divided into two main sections. The first section depicts the relationship between stress and the brain – that is, how the way that our brain works affects how we experience negative events, which ultimately leads to a feeling of stress.

In the second section, I will outline the rules that can help each of you readers to reduce the frequency of stress in your life. You will adopt a new routine with which you can better regulate your life. Also, and most importantly, you will gain skills to help you channel your feelings at extremely challenging moments. In this way, their impact on your life will be more negligible and will last far less time.

I am certain that some of my readers will be skeptical. Some of you will probably wonder how these simple recommendations will benefit you. But that is the source of their great power – the sheer simplicity and ease of implementation. For each of these steps, I will make recommendations for gradual implementation, for that is where success lies. This is a graded application that will change your lifestyle and allow you to adopt different thinking patterns.

A final tip: It is best to read the book by the sea, at sunset, with a glass of wine (not beer), and with soothing music in the background. For the "recalcitrant" among you (those who are against wine or soothing music), just breathe deeply and relax. It's all good!

WHAT IS STRESS?

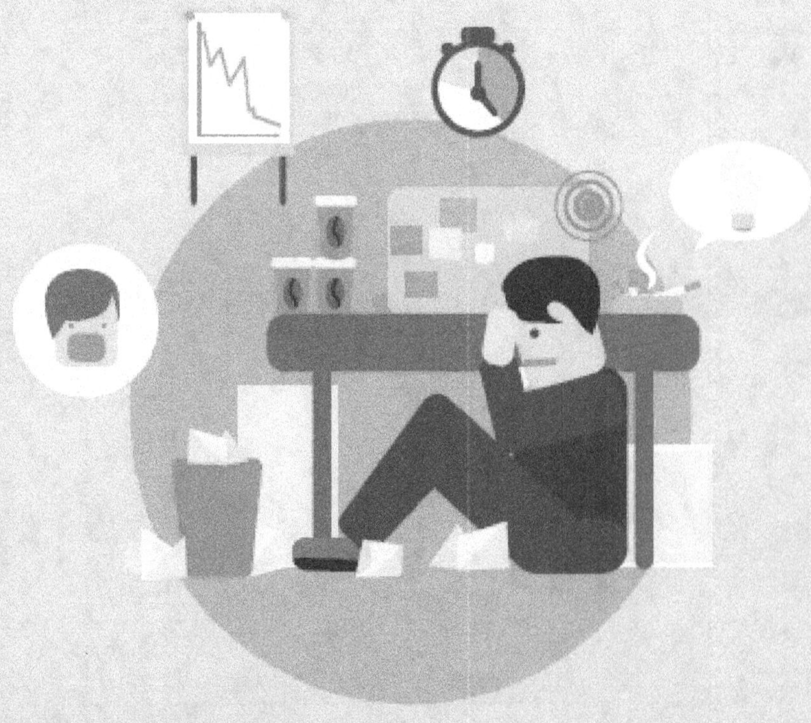

CHAPTER ONE

DEFINING STRESS

"If we are going to suffer, at least let's enjoy it."
(Folk saying)

Work is a major part of our lives, but it is also a major cause of stress…

During our adult lives, we will work more than one third of our time. The average person will spend more than seventy thousand hours at work, and others as much as one hundred twenty thousand hours. There are even those who won't stop there and will use their so-called leisure time thinking and worrying about work, time spent that is not directly defined as work hours.

Work is not performed in a vacuum. We are all in different frameworks and subject to the rules of working hours and rest. By the way, most of these rules were created decades ago, and they are not necessarily compatible with today's reality.

The title of this chapter is, "Work is a major part of our lives, but it is also a major cause of stress…" Work does indeed fill our days. It is a key factor in creating our adult persona and even allows us to fulfill our mission. At the same time, work and the workplace are major stressors, both because we stay within this framework for most of our waking hours, and also because our workplace itself presents us with quite a few challenges, most of them every single day.

Here is a little story that illustrates this. "D." is a senior level employee at a leading communications company. She approached me as an acquaintance and asked to meet. In our conversation, she told me in detail how she felt. She said she was living in a pressure cooker about to explode, and that she had already lost her taste for things that had previously given her pleasure and satisfaction at work. Every little thing caused her to become stressed, easily upset, and extremely impatient. The theme of the pressure cooker was repeated often in our conversation, accompanied by bursts of emotion that included constant crying. Indeed, I felt she was in real distress.

D. is not alone. Many people feel burnout at work, with increasing demands made upon them personally, on a group and organizational level, and even calling for national sacrifices. Many organizations, especially businesses, have become more and more demanding. In Western, developed countries there is a culture of working around the clock. Why is this so? Mainly because of the ubiquity of email, instant messaging, and the internet. We have become available and accessible without limits.

Employers require their employees to be accessible at all times. Often, this is done indirectly or covertly. Here's an example: let's say you were given a laptop with an office connection and a link for your job, as well as a smartphone with an email app. Your basic impulse will be to stay connected and up-to-date, as you are expected to have real time accessibility and availability. As a result, you may feel you have to be on call in case something unexpected may happen. Thus, your work is around the clock – it never ends.

Many people use their smartphones as an alarm clock. Imagine the following: It is midnight. You lay your head down heavily on a comfortable pillow. Suddenly, a continuous, low, vibrating sound signals the receipt of a new email. How many people do you know won't be tempted to check it out? In this kind of situation, unfortunately, we lose quite a bit of rest and certainly also compromise the very quality of our sleep.

Along with our numerous work hours, our constant availability and accessibility, there is also a feeling of insecurity in the workplace. Many employees today do not have a sense of job security. That does not necessarily mean working conditions or tenure, but rather the lack of a basic sense of stability that the employer and the workplace can provide.

The aspiration and the expectation derived from this is a culture of meeting personal and business goals. Today, we live in a corporate culture based on measurements and performance evaluation. This is a capitalistic society that values and judges people based on their position in the organizational hierarchy, their occupation, and their salary. It is this culture that creates, among other things, the sense of the absence of job security.

Fat, Forty, and *Fired: One Man's Frank, Funny,* and *Inspiring Account* of *Losing His Job* and *Finding His Life*, is a fascinating and entertaining book by Nigel Marsh.[2]

In the final chapter (which I particularly liked), the author comes to an important insight that I will try to explain briefly. For many years, Marsh explains, we have been striving for everything: a thriving career, a great family, a house in the suburbs, a new car every year, and most of all, feeling healthy and happy. Show me someone that does not dream of such things and does not strive to achieve them.

Marsh explains that life has revealed to him that we have been lied to or misled by false hopes, or at the very least, we have been given a bad recommendation. Everywhere on the globe, people are stressed more and more simply because they have failed to achieve everything they aspired to. Marsh argues that our ambition and striving for perfect balance only knocks us off balance. A perfectly balanced life is a myth, and cannot be truly achieved.

Does Marsh recommend that we all give up? He claims not to do so. He simply advises us not to be stressed because we have not achieved everything we wished for: amazing careers, wonderful children, and most of all, work-family balance. There is also a gray area; not everything in life is black or white. We just have to tell ourselves that life is hard and most likely will always be hard. That acknowledgement itself is a great relief.

One can dispute Marsh's conclusions, but we can also draw an important conclusion of our own: setting a goal of achieving perfect balance in life is a double-edged sword that can further nurture the imbalance. When we strive to achieve balance in life, we must realize that from a practical point of view, we have no control over all the factors involved.

Instead of setting a goal that will undoubtedly be difficult to achieve and even increase feelings of stress, eventually bringing you to burnout, let us make simple, small, every day decisions that are easy to achieve. For example, instead of setting ourselves the goal of spending more time with the children, we simply decide that on a specific day we will come home earlier from work and spend a pleasant hour or so with them. Instead of deciding that we are not answering any emails after six o'clock, we will just decide that today, while we are spending time with the children, we will not answer the phone, do any work on the computer, or read any emails.

Burnout is not the subject of this book, but it was important for me to focus on it to illustrate the connection between burnout and stress. Burnout is indeed one of the causes of stress, but it is also nourished by it and there exists a Gordian knot between these two factors.

So…What the Devil is Demon Stress?

The origin of the word "stress" is from the Latin "Strictus," which means "drawn tight." Synonyms for stress are: pressure, tension, and strain.

Initially, the term was used in the field of fiscal science, primarily to define a given situation where one object is projected onto another. Over the years, the term has also been adopted by other scientific fields, such as the medical sciences. Stress in the eyes of medicine is a necessary and even essential response of the body to a change in our environment. The term is also used in social sciences and ordinary vernacular.

Stress is prominent in the workplace as well. Organizations

today face many complex challenges, including increased competition, business globalization, rapid technological advancement, employees demanding higher wages and rewards, and better working conditions, the power of unions, and various other pressure groups.

Employees themselves need to develop and expand their knowledge, to become more educated and professional, and function effectively in an environment full of new technologies that are developing at lightning speed. They are expected to improve their efficiency and effectiveness as well as their overall functioning, and work under challenging conditions, often in different languages and with different cultures.

Management is on one hand employees of the organization, so they face the same challenges as any regular employee, but as leaders they are required to both meet the organization's requirements and supervise their employees. In fact, they are required to be responsible for a great many things, and almost all of them need to be dealt with at the same time.

In general, we feel stress when we perceive that we have no control over what happens to us in our lives, so stress usually has a negative connotation for us. When this occurs, we sense the gap between what we want to happen and what actually does happen. The brain sees this as a threat that can affect our mental state as well as our physical equilibrium.

Stress is not a new phenomenon. Even in ancient times people felt tension and sadness, but in those times the scale of sensations was different and a deterioration in the "quality of life" was not a trigger for stress.

If I was destined to live a life of economic hardship, so be it. That fact in itself did not make me anxious. Today, the range of comfort available and our aspiration for a high level quality of life, which is expressed mainly in material possessions, our global exposure on social networks, our tendency to measure everything with a subjective measure of the "quality of life." often creates a feeling of frustration. We are increasingly aware of what a "comfortable" life can offer us and attaining it becomes a key factor in our lives.

Stress is an important component in our lives and will always be present, but it also has positive aspects, as we shall see below. The secret of how to deal effectively with it is its power and frequency. It is also important to understand that stress, or rather the way we perceive stress, is not objective. The symptoms are, of course, objective and they are measurable and treatable, but the feeling itself is subjective and influenced by our unique personal experiences, our backgrounds, and personality traits.

It is difficult to define stress precisely and unequivocally, but it can be said that what is common to all definitions of stress is that it affects us mentally and is sometimes accompanied by detrimental physical, emotional, and social symptoms.

Often the pressure that creates the stress arises, owing to the difference between a person's expectations of himself or those around him, and the actual situation as it exists in reality.

It is important to note that stress is not linked to temporary or short-term pressures. Most of us know how to deal with temporary situations. Stress is usually linked to a long-lasting condition. How long? There is no exact timetable, but in my opinion, a few weeks or more is enough time to bring about stress. What are the most influential factors that create this pressure? Many studies in this area have found that stressors can be divided into several categories:

Everyday Difficulties – These are usually not very significant, but in some cases they can be troublesome and cause a growing feeling of tension. For example, having to get up early to prepare breakfast, pack lunches, take the children to kindergarten or school, get stuck in traffic, and arrive at work at the very last minute. This is certainly an everyday hassle most of us go through and it ought not to be overly serious, but at certain times and in some situations it can cause great frustration and tension, and act as a stressor.

Feelings of Frustration – Frustration is an emotional state we feel particularly when we are unable to meet a goal or a given task. It is a negative feeling that becomes stronger as the gap between the goal and the outcome increases or is affected by the emotional importance connected to achieving the goal and our motivation to accomplish it. For example, suppose we set ourselves the goal of getting a promotion at work. We applied for a higher position but we were not chosen. In many cases, this is definitely a source of frustration. Other situations at work that can produce frustration are: actual job loss, the threat of dismissal, substantial changes in the organization, job change, and more.

Conflict – Conflict is a common situation where we are required to choose between two or more alternatives that are often different from one another. For example, in the case of women who are mothers of young children, there is a frequent, ongoing conflict between work and family. The degree of complexity of the conflict, the amount of time spent on it, and how difficult it will be to choose one or the other will determine whether this particular conflict becomes one that causes stress.

Life Changes – Significant life changes can be a major stress factor. Examples: Dealing with the loss of a family member or close friend, dismissal from work, or even positive changes such as moving house, pregnancy, childbirth, marriage, etc.

Employment Factors – These can be divided into two subgroups:

1. Occupation Characteristics. Examples: High job demands, job mismatch, job uncertainty and ambiguity, staff responsibilities social life or job tasks, job load, role image, routine versus dynamic issues, and intensive working conditions.

2. Characteristics of the Organization. Examples: Long working hours, shift work, job insecurity, lack of job control, social isolation in the workplace, corporate unfairness and injustice, exposure to prejudice, racism, and/or sexual harassment.

3. Dramatic Events in the Environment – Dramatic events that occur in our immediate surroundings, or even distant ones can be a trigger for stress. Examples: Natural disasters such as COVID 19 pandemic, hurricanes, dealing with huge fires, war, or political crises.

Coping with stress usually starts in the brain. The brain, through one of the five senses, receives a danger signal and prepares to deal with the threat, usually by a "fight response, freeze, or flight." It is a mechanism inherent in man from the earliest times, but in the modern age this mechanism is often triggered for no reason and in situations that do not justify a fight or flight response because they are not life-threatening.

When stressed, we experience various symptoms that can be divided into different categories:

- **Immediate Physical Reactions** – such as accelerating heart rate, a rise in blood pressure (both systolic and diastolic), increasing muscle tension, increased sweating,
- Acceleration of the respiratory rate, change in brain electrical activity and increased secretion of adrenaline. Also, a person in a state of mental stress is more exposed to mild illnesses such as colds, allergies, chronic muscle pain, and even more serious illnesses such as hypertension, heart disease, or gastrointestinal disorders such as bowel disorders, Crohn's disease, and Colitis.
- **Mental Reactions** – In many cases people who experience stress report a decrease in concentration and memory, as well as a reduction in attention and errors in judgment.
- **Emotional Reactions** – This category includes anxiety or depression as well as feelings of distress and sadness.

- **Behavioral Delays** – One of the consequences of stress is the effect on the person's overt behavior. This can be reflected in violent outbursts, verbal outrage, physical reactions, aggression, withdrawal, and an increase in negative habits, such as cigarette smoking, alcohol consumption, and drug abuse.

With the help of this book, you will learn what causes stress, what are the mechanisms in the brain that control it, and more importantly, you will learn the skills to enable you to neutralize and reduce the brain's automatic responses when it recognizes distress.

The main idea behind this method, which I will elaborate on later in the book, is training the brain and the body to cope with stress. The training focuses on recognition and awareness. The goal of training is to make sure that in moments of stress we become fully attentive to our feelings, and we are able to replace old, bad habits with new, positive ones.

The book focuses on in-depth knowledge of the subject and presents it in a simple, absorbing manner, so that with daily, long-term practice we can live with stress and not allow it to so powerfully take over our lives.

In recent years, many studies have pointed to the important role of cognitive factors in situations of stress in humans. As a scientific term, stress is actually a response to a stimulus that causes an increase in the level of arousal of the brain. This is a process where there is a stimulus and there is a response to the stimulus.

In fact, the physiological response will be the same whether our assessment of results is positive or negative, which of course is based on our life experience and our innate expectations.

Let us suppose that I am currently competing for a coveted position and rumor has it that my competition for the position is an extremely talented person whom I have long feared. In this case, the initial stimulus is the rumor, and the response is my negative interpretation of the stimulus.

Ursin and Eriksen presented a model called "*Cognitive Activation Theory of Stress*"[3] (CATS for short).

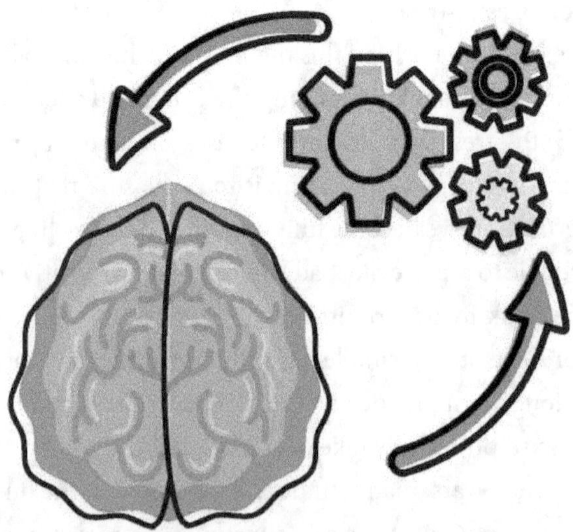

The emotional load or weight is created as a result of stimuli or stressors. This emotional load is measured by the brain in a process that we are not aware of at all, and as a result, the brain may classify this condition as a threat alert. Our response to this alert (the physiological response alongside the psychological response) will be a reflexive response to the stimulus and will depend on many individual characteristics such as our personality, life experience, past traumas, etc.

If the alert is classified as negative, the emotional weight over time will become stressful. It is important to understand that the way we respond the first time to the stimulus that created the stress becomes a pattern, and the brain will act the same way in similar circumstances. The pattern is complicated to explain. Let's just say it becomes a behavioral pattern.

The brain can classify a particular situation as a threat (negative), but it can also classify it as a challenge (positive). The brain is an efficient organ and it operates with psychological evaluation and processing of our behavior. The threat alert will be activated in our minds when there is a large gap between what we hope will happen and what happens in reality.

I was recently contacted by an acquaintance of mine who told me about an employee of hers. This same employee had fainted several times and as a result all of her workmates were debating how to behave with her and were on edge. After an inquiry her employee went through, it turned out she was suffering from anxiety attacks that had recently begun to affect her, for no apparent reason. This same employee asked herself, "What is happening to me? How did this suddenly happen? After all, I have never suffered these attacks before." My acquaintance who is the supervisor of this employee discreetly asked her to see her family doctor and ask him for advice.

The employee felt frightened, aimless, and filled with

exhausting questions and thoughts. She said she avoided going out of her home alone for fear of a sudden anxiety attack. This happens often, even though sometimes the original stimulus that brought on the alarm in our brain is gone, we are still preoccupied with the fear of an anxiety attack.

Many studies on this issue have pointed this out as the main consequence of anxiety attacks. The desire for avoidance and the fear of the fear itself, a dread of the unpleasantness that I may experience.

However, the discrepancy between the outcome we had hoped for and what actually happens can serve as a catalyst for increasing our motivation. It involves the same mechanism in the brain that can either cause stress or excite motivation. The difference lies in our interpretation of the discrepancy between our aspirations and what really happens.

Take tennis, for example. Note the actions of the players on the court. When Player A hits the ball, Player B moves quickly toward where he thinks the ball will land. How does he know? After all, he doesn't have time to sit down and analyze the situation. The brain works instantaneously in the same way. Once a stimulus is created, the complex system, based in part on our senses, quickly absorbs the information, analyzes it, and, based on past actions, guides our bodies to move in the expected direction where the ball will land.

The anticipation of events by the brain is an important key to how it works – based on gathering, processing, and storing information for a specific stimulus. In essence, the brain teaches us by embedding the information within us as well as performing the same basic processes that include information about the stimulus itself – how it was classified previously and how we behaved in the past when it was activated. If we go back to the tennis game, the brain is expecting the hit ball to trigger the same reactions as in previous cases.

Choosing to deal with stress is the best strategy to regulate its effect. Coping allows the brain to classify stress alerts more positively: "You can handle this," "It won't kill me," "All these problems have a solution." Over time, our coping will reduce the brain's arousal for threat situations. What matters in this theory is taking action, the choice to deal with it. This is an important point, as the result itself is less important. It is less important if we are able to reduce stress or not…what is more important is the action we have taken, our choice to cope rather than repress or avoid the stress.

Try this little experiment. List at least one thing you habitually avoid. For starters, you can choose something small, but it still must be something that bothers you and makes you tense. Choose to take action and deal with it. You will find that neither the result nor the feedback you receive are what matters, but your subjective sense that you have succeeded in coping. You will definitely feel that your response to stress has changed for the better.

The strategies I outline in the last chapters of the book include ways to deal with stress. The guiding principle is to cope as long as you can, and to take defensive action only when you have to.

That is, it is advisable that you protect yourself in a situation where you perceive a tangible and imminent danger, such as a lion in the jungle coming after you, or a truck that is speeding toward you at maximum speed. As long as these extreme situations are not the case, you can choose to cope with the stress.

Keeping things in proportions is very important as not all stress or pressure are necessarily dangerous. Dealing with stress to minimize its harmfulness will prevent deleterious long-term effects, as doing nothing to cope with chronic stress can endanger your health and diminish your quality of life.

CHAPTER TWO

IT'S ALL IN YOUR HEAD – THE BRAIN AND STRESS

"Life is what happens to you while you're busy making other plans." (**John Lennon,** Beautiful Boy)

The human brain is a machine, a tool, a system, and an organism of unimaginable complexity. One can say with certainty that there is a great deal more unknown than is known about how it works from current research. Compared to other elements in nature, the power of its causality, and analytic ability are strongest in the human brain. How does the brain work? What are the mechanisms that trigger, control, and regulate stress? These are the key questions that we will attempt to answer extensively in this chapter.

I wrote the chapter so that on one hand it would describe as accurately as possible the structure of the brain and the central processes that take place within it, and on the other hand I have tried to write it in plain language so that any functioning person could understand it.

The Structure of the Brain

The brain is the central organ in our nervous system and it controls, activates, and monitors everything we feel, the way we think, and behave. Brain research is a field that has been increasingly evolving in recent years and is a magnet for researchers in many different fields of endeavor.

We channel and process information, consciously and unconsciously with the brain. Information, which is essentially sensory, is transmitted to the nerve cells. Any information absorbed through our senses is "translated" into the brain by neural conduction and then for changes in the biological function of the cells, carrying messages to the target organ.

The brain is encased within the skull and wrapped in membranes. It is linked through the peripheral nervous system to the spinal cord, which is the main conduit to the rest of the body's organs.

The Structure of the Human Brain Consists of Three Sections: The Cerebrum ("big brain"), the Brainstem, and the Cerebellum ("little brain").

The Cerebrum, the largest section of the brain, is responsible for the bulk of sensory information processing and the transfer of commands for voluntary actions.

The brain stem is the thread that connects the brain to the spine and is responsible, among other things, for transporting sensory information.

The cerebellum is the "operations manager" that enables the coordination of motor activity.

Cerebrum (big brain)

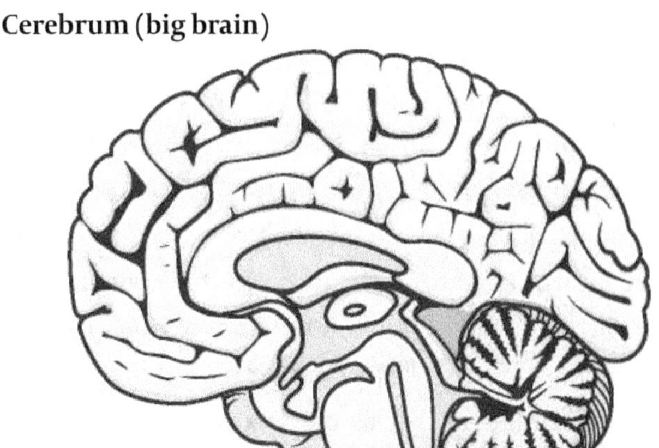

Cerebellum (little brain)

The Cerebrum, or big brain, is the section that interests us most, as it is the one that links emotions with behavior. The four elements that control our emotional and behavioral responses to stress are located in the big brain and are called the amygdala, hypothalamus, hippocampus, and anterior cortex.

The Amygdala

The amygdala takes up a very small area in the brain (a little more than one inch) with an almond-like shape. It consists of thirteen nuclei and is located at the depth of the middle retinal lobe of our brain. Sounds like Chinese? I imagine so, but the following sentences will make things clear.

My way of remembering the amygdala's role and weird name is to simply ascribe to it some meaning. I visualize the amygdala as a watchtower with ultra-sensitive sensors that are activated when the brain is in a waking state.

Incidentally, memories from the time of our birth to age three are mostly stored in this deep part of the brain and this is probably the reason, to our good fortune, that we do not remember almost anything from this period in our lives.

The amygdala operates as a watchtower, equipped with our main alarm system. It is responsible for regulating the action of the hormonal and autonomic nervous systems. The amygdala absorbs sensory information from the environment and immediately classifies it, determining whether the information is emotionally important to us.

The amygdala functions as an emotional link to fear processes. When the amygdala senses something it categorizes as a threat, it immediately and automatically activates the emotional alarm system and transmits to the hypothalamus (the watchtower security officer) to prepare the body for a response.

This is why we may feel our heart rate accelerating even before we are consciously aware of a threat. Take, for example, a situation where your attention is focused on your computer monitor, and suddenly behind you, without your knowing, someone claps their hands loudly. Even before you can decide what to do, your brain will be on emergency alert and your immediate response will be a surprised shout and a startled jump accompanied by an accelerated heartbeat.

What I have just described is a situation where stress stimulation (stressor) is triggered. In this instance, much of our brain's resources will be directed to the threat or emergency situation that the brain has identified and the body will enter into a state of alert.

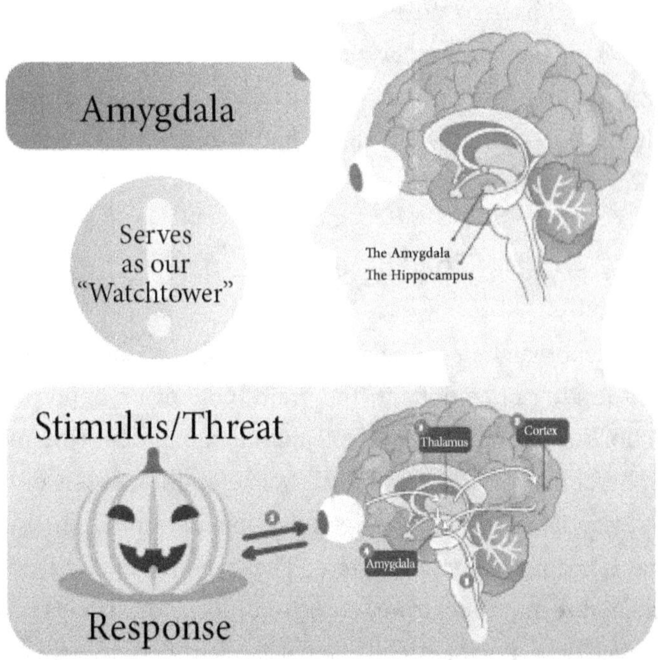

The amygdala is involved in other functions linked to cognition, including attention, study, and associative learning. The amygdala is one of the most interconnected areas of the brain and its location as a central emotional region allows it to integrate and disseminate information to many other parts of the brain, including those that support cognitive functions.

Another interesting fact is that the amygdala is responsible for the emotional aspect of memory, which means that the amygdala also links the information we have received through the senses and takes it to an emotional dimension such as anger, disappointment, joy, or sadness. In this way, a cognitive-value meaning is linked to the experience.

Let's go back to the loud clapping of hands I mentioned earlier. If the surprise event is repeated several times, the amygdala is likely to cause us to turn our heads around almost every time we sit down and focus our eyes on the computer screen.

The Hypothalamus

The hypothalamus is the area responsible for coordinating and linking operations in the brain. One of its important actions is the activation of the autonomic system (the peripheral nervous system that allows autonomous activation of essential actions, such as circulation and respiration) and the hormone secretion system. The hypothalamus can be likened to the watchtower security officer, who is currently receiving a signal. If the signal is identified as a threat, the hypothalamus will automatically operate according to a pre-existing pattern.

A pressure alert is first acquired by the amygdala. The "security officer" in the hypothalamus then works to provide the needed resources to deal with the threat. In other words, the hypothalamus is responsible for activating the hormonal system required to deal with the threat and for secreting specific hormones into our bloodstream. At the end of the process, when the brain defines the state of stress, hormones such as cortisol prepare our bodies to cope with the stressor. (For example, our capacity for fight or flight.)

The Hippocampus

The hippocampus reminds many people of a sea horse. It can be likened to the knowledge manager of the system, acting as a skilled librarian and cataloging vast amounts of information that come from many different sources. Like any knowledge system, the secret is in its method of extracting and cataloging the information.

The library itself (or the archive) is located in the frontal cortex. This part of the brain is responsible for the storage and retrieval of long-term conscious memories associated with certain situations. The hippocampus also plays an important role in the creation of new conscious memories. Conscious memories mean memories that can be associated with a particular space, place, time, or people, and most importantly, they can be expressed in words.

In pressure situations, the hippocampus helps to link the causes of the current stress state with similar past events that are stored in memory. For example, if we try to bring to mind a stressful event we experienced in our past, such as a car accident we were involved in, we can recover from that memory how we reacted and what the results were of those reactions.

Utilizing these memories (and understanding their context) is essential to humans as thinking beings. It enables us to learn for the future and is a central element of our benefitting from past mistakes or past experiences in general. Often, momentary stresses can cause the hippocampus to be inactive and the amygdala to operate instead. This is a situation where the "knowledge manager" did not function and the "security officer" took control without having the processing and knowledge ability that our expert knowledge manager has.

In such cases we may be able to resolve the threat, but the event that caused the stress and our reactions to it will not be stored in the brain, and the next time a similar event occurs, the brain will react without recalling the desired responses. Therefore, in more ongoing stressful situations, it is useful to have the brain engage our knowledge manager and not let the security officer handle it. That way the brain can more effectively process the event and its reactions and results. The next time the brain can react with an appropriate response, as the event catalog will allow it to identify and retrieve the most correct action and response pattern, which have been successful in the past.

Now I would like you to close your eyes for a moment and try to remember a situation at work that causes you fear. Many senior executives are troubled by periodic board meetings. This trepidation is often accompanied by unpleasant physical sensations, such as breaking out in a cold sweat and heart palpitations. Many try to cope with these feelings by telling themselves that this is another ongoing, scheduled meeting. However, if participation in other meetings has been perceived as intimidating, even if this is not an emotional fact, it is highly likely that they will experience the same uneasiness and sense of pressure before every meeting of this type.

Let's try to analyze what is going on in our minds before the board meeting. First, our brain elicits a similar memory from the past and creates a link between the upcoming board meeting and the emotions experienced at previous board meetings. The link causes a physical reaction to a condition that the brain categorizes as threatening.

Because our brains have categorized the event as negative, we have pulled out the most appropriate response. What can we do to change it? Quite a bit, it turns out…but that we will see in the coming chapters.

The Prefrontal Cortex

The cortex is the area of the brain that surrounds the outer layer of the Cerebrum, the large brain. The cortex is the element that manages and organizes the information and the necessary actions to be taken. The cortex is also responsible for processing sensory information into conscious, cognitive and motor activity. Many refer to it as the CEO, or "the brains" of the organization.

This section of the brain facilitates a conscious link between the information processed in the amygdala and hippocampus and the subsequent action required in response to a stress situation. The prefrontal cortex, or anterior prefrontal cortex as it is sometimes called, receives information from other regions of the brain and integrates it all, thus directing our overall behavior. Equally interesting is the fact that the cortex is also involved in the diagnosis of our mood as well as that of others. This is possible because the cortex's activities are aimed at, among other things, the creation of mental images of the world. The reading of a thought is actually the visual image of our thoughts, our feelings, and our beliefs.

Responses to stress that will be managed by the frontal

cortex will be more conscious, calculated and linked to learning from past events. For example, in dealing with a stressful situation such as a job assessment meeting with a direct superior, the cortex reminds us of how much good work we did this year, and that all in all, the conversation in the previous year was quite pleasant and helpful. This will relax the amygdala's involvement in the process, and reduce the stress response to the current event, as it may no longer be perceived as a major stressor.

As we proceed, we will learn a technique that will allow us to quickly catalog events in such a way that the "CEO" can operate without active involvement of the "watchtower security officer," so we can lower the "voltage" of the alarm system.

The Flexible Brain

In 2007, psychiatrist Dr. Norman Doidge[4] published a comprehensive book called, *The Brain that Changes Itself.* In his book, Doidge presented extensive research from many independent sources in the field of brain research. All the studies had one common conclusion: that the brain is an organic, flexible organ, and contrary to what we had previously thought, it is capable of being repaired.

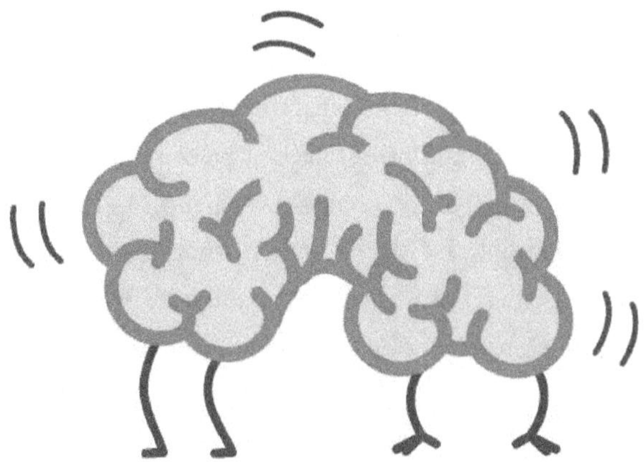

It was recently reported that an Italian neurosurgeon, Professor Sergio Canavero, is conducting a series of studies that have led to a scientific breakthrough and has even been tested on animals. Canavero came to the conclusion that one person's head could be transplanted onto another person's body. For now, this seems like science is fiction at best, or at worst, the ravings of a mad, unethical professor who is merely seeking sensationalism and notoriety. However you perceive Canavero's claim, scientific research is convinced that there is no need for brain transplants, as our brain and the way important processes operate within it can be altered.

The brain is a living, dynamic, and changing organ. It adapts to the events and memories that we humans experience. The mind is resilient and evolves throughout our lives in sync with the experiences we go through at every stage of our lives. The transformation of the brain as a result of our individual experiences is not only neural or emotional but structural, so much so that research has shown that new genes are created in the nerve cells of the brain.

It turns out that people are indeed different and unique, even though we are all born with the same set of tools (for example, the skeletal and muscular system or sensory system.)

Humans have five senses: sight, hearing, taste, smell, and touch. In his book, Doidge[4] explains that our senses should be treated as smart power converters that transforms energy through motion or pressure into electrical energy that flows into our nerve cells. This is how the brain perceives the world around us.

If we think of a threatening situation such as fear, our brain has an immediate response switch with three states: fight, fright, or freeze. When the switch is turned on, the brain, through our sensors, turns off most of the areas that are not needed to focus the energy and resources of the brain to deal with the situation with one of the three states.

The perception of the brain as a flexible, repairable, organ is interesting in and of itself. Many of us choose to describe how the brain works from concepts taken from the world of computers or machines. We tend to treat the brain as a CPU or as a complex, even "perfect" machine. Using such conceptions gives the brain a certain structure with different connected parts, each one with a role, but this does not reflect its flexibility.

The flexible brain that can change itself as described by Doidge alters the way we perceive the brain and associated images. Conceiving of the brain as a living and continually evolving organ means that it is possible to retrain and reshape it. The brain consists of malleable, linkable parts that can operate independently but also depend on each other. Every part has a defined role, but it also has the ability to process different types of input. This allows the brain to evolve and be susceptible to influences over the years, even throughout adulthood.

One of the variables that can affect the ability to process information in the brain is being in a high-intensity environment. A stimulus-rich environment allows for higher learning capability than an environment where there are not many stimuli. In animal experiments, it was found that when animals were in the presence of many stimuli, the weight of the cerebral cortex increased and so did the size and number of connections between the nerve cells. The cells grew significantly and the blood supply to them increased[4]. These, and other findings, have led to the new image of the brain as a muscle that grows and develops as you continue to train it.

It is important to note that there are also quite a few processes in the brain that can be spoken of as conscious processes, i.e., they are a function of information processing and decision making. Such processes often occur in a nanosecond. Automated processes are essential for us to work efficiently. Think of what life would be if every morning when we got out of bed we would have to start to think how to get up and where to go. In actuality, most of our daily operations are automatic and eventually become acquired habits.

There are many physical activities such as eating, breathing, or driving, that we simply know how to do. We always know more than we are aware of. This knowledge is often called "covert knowledge" and it allows us to assimilate an activity that we have habitually practiced so that it becomes fully automatic without our being conscious of it.

The processes of the brain that are not automatic are instances where a conscious decision has to be made, to study or to speak with a friend. These are processes that are consciously controlled and involve many areas of the brain. To illustrate this, take the following situation:

Sit with a friend and show him that you're not in a good mood. Do not smile throughout the meeting and use terms such as "not easy," "hard day," "very, very busy," "I have no desire for anything," etc. Later on, after you part company, ask your friend to describe how the rest of his day went. There's a good chance he'll tell you it wasn't one of his better days. Why does he respond that way?

It often turns out that unconsciously absorbed information (the non-smiling face, the rigid body language) causes an automatic response. Your friend did not make any conscious decision to be affected by your behavior, he is simply not able to control his reaction (it is controlled automatically by his brain). Some researchers call this process the "cognitive unconscious"[5].

So we can see now that we are influenced by factors not necessarily under our control, just as you saw that the mood of your friend was affected by your mood without his or her being aware of it. We tend to think that we act out of free will, but it turns out that is not always the case. The good news is that the brain can certainly be taught to control responses through practice and focus. It is important that we understand that we respond to the emotions of others around us and adapt our own emotions accordingly.

When we meet with an acquaintance and ask how he

is feeling, we are opening ourselves up to possibly hearing a sob story about the difficult times our friend is going through. This will inevitably affect the way we are feeling. There will be those of us who get into our cars after hearing the difficulties someone else is going through and tell themselves that they should be happy with their own lives, and how important it is to see things in proportion after such a sad encounter with their friend.

There will be others who will be affected differently and they will have to recover from the stressful meeting for hours. Whatever way you respond to the story, what is clear is that your feelings will be influenced by your personal interpretation of what your friend has revealed to you.

Another important distinction lies in the perception of the flexible brain. I will introduce this by telling you of a personal experience. In a conversation with my fifteen-year-old daughter who doesn't like to read books, I tried to convince her how important it is to read but the bored look on her face said it all, "Dad you're old-fashioned, you don't have to read books anymore, today you can listen to podcasts or download audio books instead!"

If we take the case of listening to books versus reading them, then according to the perception of the flexible brain not only is the content (the words) important, but also the medium that delivers them. (For example, reading or listening.) It is a different concept than in the past, when a word was processed in an area of the brain that assimilates and understands written words.

In an interesting study conducted in 2001, by research groups at Carnegie Mellon University, precisely this issue was examined. The researchers[6] found that different areas of the brain processed the input from listening. Not only that, they also showed that there are different centers of understanding of the word depending whether it is read or heard. That means that listening to a book will leave us with different memories than reading the same book.

The Flexible Mind is not merely a concept, it is also a branch of science that believes that in-depth research can lead to a better understanding not only of how the brain functions, but also how the brain can be influenced, trained, and ultimately shaped to affect the way we live.

The Foggy Brain

The foggy brain is a term used by cognitive experts. It refers to those situations in which we are often, and for extended periods of time, disturbed by piercingly negative thoughts. Psychologically, the foggy brain is on the borderline between mental health and chronic illness, such as anxiety, depression, and even feelings of utter hopelessness.

In recent years, alarming data has been published about our mental state. In a 2018 Mental Health America report, it is estimated that one out of five adult Americans (about 40 million people!) reported a state of mind that was not optimal in their perception, and only a fraction of them turned to a professional for help. In Western culture, it can, therefore, be said with great confidence that a great many of us are probably in this situation. What I mean is that many of us are not in an optimal state of mind, yet nevertheless we will not seek professional help.

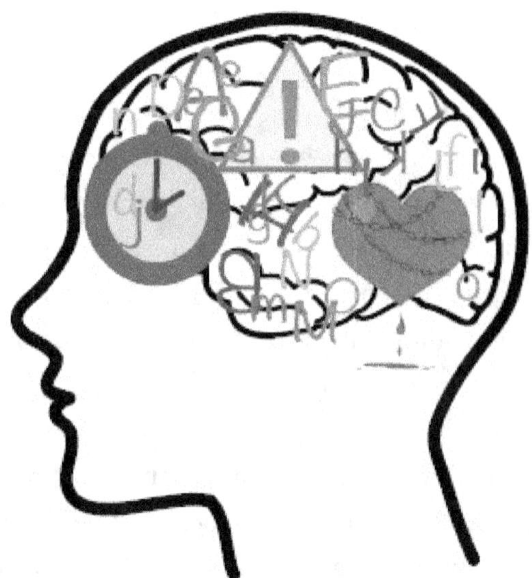

Here is a personal example. Every Saturday night my feelings are different from my feelings during the week. On Sunday night, my thoughts start to wander in all different directions. I think of the presentation I failed to make, the urgent emails I haven't answered, important meetings coming up, and the smart answers everyone expects me to come up with. On Mondays, I am always more tired and moodier than usual.

Why is this? Outwardly, I'm supposed to be satisfied and relaxed. The weekend was successful, family fun, sports, rest. You would think I would feel great on Monday morning. But that is not the case. It turns out that not only do I feel this way, but also many others do. Mondays are stressful because most everyone comes back to work in this same frame of mind as in the Boomtown Rats song, "I don't like Mondays."

By comparison, Friday is my favorite day. On Friday I feel focused, vital, and in high spirits. Does that mean I don't like my job and my work? Absolutely not. I feel very satisfied working in a meaningful job, but I seem to suffer like we all live on the border between an optimal state of mind and one that is not optimal. Apparently I'm in a mental state of distraction or fogginess. When the brain is foggy, it's likely to be unbalanced, sometimes feeling light, sometimes heavy, depending on different levels of hormones, including those responsible for our emotional state – serotonin, dopamine, and cortisol.

Serotonin affects feelings of serenity, optimism, and self-confidence. Dopamine is responsible for feelings such as elation, positive excitement, and satisfaction. Cortisol is the stress hormone and is secreted in stressful states. The desired state is where there is a chemical balance in the brain. Thus, it is clear that when there is even a slight hormonal imbalance we feel hazy and this will have an effect on our behavior.

I have been recently following statements made by Israeli Prime Minister Benjamin Netanyahu. Netanyahu is undisputedly a man who knows how to use the media for his own purposes. When he was recently accused of criminal activity, no matter what was asked of him, he would give a brief reply, almost always without responding to the charges or to what was being asked.

His message was short and catchy, "Nothing will come of it because there was nothing." He does as his counterpart in America, President Donald Trump does, etching it into the minds of his supporters that the media is dredging up so-called "false facts."

Research has shown that if something is repeated over and over, even though it is inaccurate, people will come to believe it, no matter how the information was presented, when, and by whom. This is a creation of a true illusion created by a memory illusion.

Try it yourself. State something with great fervor and as sincerely as you can, and if you have a credible reputation, I assure you that not only will your listeners believe it, but so will you!

Another characteristic of the brain is the different intensity of the negative emotional experience compared to the positive emotional experience. I recently went out with my partner for a relaxed dinner and told her that I had been promoted and that I was happy. Of course we both were. However, when we got back home I discovered I had forgotten my wallet at the restaurant. Desperate phone calls and searches all over did not help, the wallet had disappeared… not to mention one thousand dollars in cash and an important note I had in it, which had emotional significance for me.

Unfortunately, the brain is more affected by negative information than positive information. The distress I felt at losing my wallet was much more powerful than the elation I felt from my promotion at work. This is because of the activity of the amygdala.

As we explained earlier, when something very unpleasant happens, the brain immediately goes into action, treating it as an emergency and the buttons are pushed: fight, flight, or freeze.

If we experience the event as negative, we will continue to process it long after it is over.

The mind tends to use this negative information as part of its evolutionary development for survival by guarding against the worst of it. Given this fact, it is important that we be aware that there is something we can do – even the neurotics among us. If we train our brains to deal with negative events with a more positive interpretation of the event, then slowly we can balance the intensity of the negative with the intensity of the positive.

A positive interpretation that can be associated with an event, at first perceived as negative or threatening, is sometimes called a "re-evaluation." We can re-evaluate the event we experienced and look at it from a different angle.

For example, suppose you receive a letter from the IRS asking you to send them a full list of your capital assets. Usually when you open the mailbox and see an envelope with the income tax logo, the amygdala, which is responsible for the rapid processing of fear, anxiety, and other kinds of negative emotions leaps into action. If, at that moment, you were having an MRI or your blood pressure taken, you would certainly see an increase in amygdala activity along with a rise in blood pressure.

With reassessment of a situation, we make it more positive. We can tell ourselves that it does not have to be a threatening situation and that we might open the letter and find out it is just a standard form letter.

When we emphasize the positive aspects of the experience we can change our attitude. In this sense, the phrase "thought-creating reality" is quite true. Thoughts can change our way of thinking and enable us to perceive the reality around us in a less negative, more positive way.

Reassessment is not a tool based on an in-depth factual analysis. It is a cognitive tool. The thought is not the fact itself, but how we perceive the fact. When we reassess a situation we transfer control in the brain from the amygdala to the anterior brain regions, such as the cortex. Involving the cortex allows the amygdala to step aside for a moment, and allow us to consciously process the experience. From a threat status, we can move to a new analysis of the situation. Sometimes, conscious analysis will allow us to regulate our initial emotional response – in other words, to re-assess.

The essential act is the reassessment. The content and content analysis are less important. I will try to clarify this. Often, when we experience a negative event our brain labels it as that, according to our initial impression. In the case where we receive a letter with the IRS logo, merely seeing the letter created within us an initial classification by the amygdala that it was a threat.

The experience of processing is subconsciously affected by previous, similar perceptions. We may have recently read an article about the negative aspects of the power of the tax authorities and the fact that people have been detained, arrested, questioned, and charged due to issues with the authorities. This unconscious memory creates the same negative effect as the letter we received, regardless of its content, which is unknown to us until we open it.

If we can consciously identify the emotion we are experiencing, such as fear, anxiety, or sadness, it will create a cognitive labeling of the emotion. Research shows that such emotional labeling diminishes the intensity of our reaction to it. Why is this?

Labeling emotions activates the anterior regions of the brain[7] (where linguistic processing is carried out, among other things), and the brain balances the sensations by reducing the activity of the amygdala. This can reduce the power of a long-term emotional response. In this way, we actually regulate brain function, so the next time we receive a letter from the IRS, the intensity of our initial response will be much less and most likely not as stressful.

Reassessment is a more effective way of emotional regulation (or as it is called in everyday language "self-control.") Research shows that emotional regulation can actually produce the opposite reaction in us from what it was intended to produce.

Emotional regulation accompanies us in everyday life, enabling us to adhere to the rules of the society in which we live. For example, we learn that it is not always necessary to express anger when we feel it. Society at large encourages restraint and self-control.

Emotional regulation in stressful situations can lead to an uncomfortable mood and lower functioning because it is a process that requires a great deal of effort, one that depletes the mental energy resources we require. In contrast, emotional labeling through linguistic processing can have a positive long-term effect, especially when labeling and processing are carried out very soon after the occurrence of the negative experience[8]

PART TWO

THE EFFECTS OF STRESS IN OUR LIVES

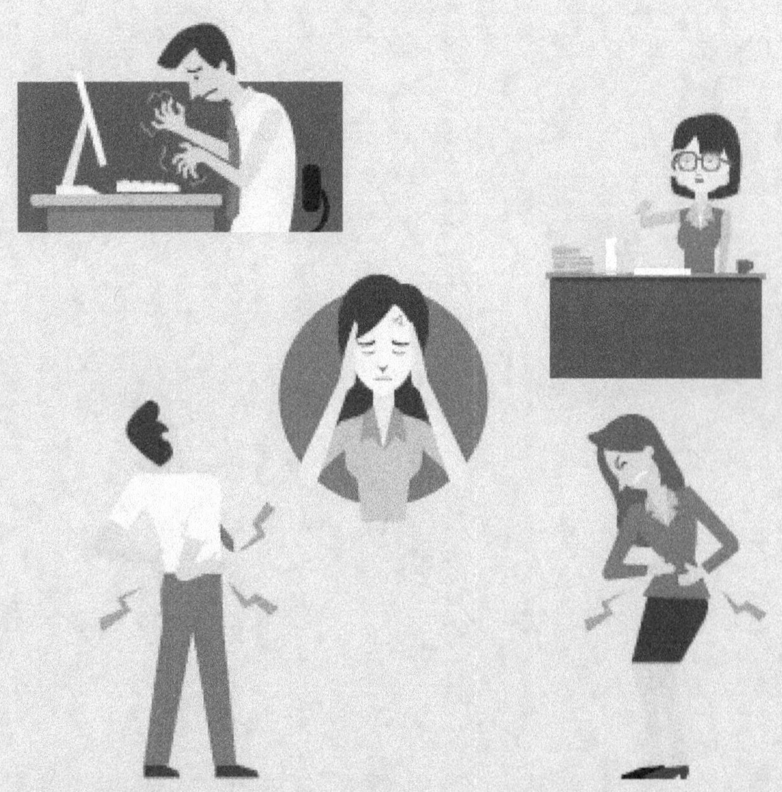

CHAPTER THREE

THE EFFECTS OF STRESS IN OUR LIVES

"I'm not afraid of death, I just don't want to be there when it happens." (**Woody Allen**)

"A.," in her early forties, is a senior manager at an international company. Ostensibly she leads an enjoyable life with a successful marriage and children. Recently, A. began suffering from severe back pain. The pains came on sporadically and randomly.

"My back went out again," her family heard the complaint time after time. "I can't move, I can't get out of bed."

Comprehensive diagnostic tests did not show anything out of the ordinary except a slipped disc, a minor nuisance that many people suffer from.

A., however, continued to suffer from pain that caused her severe distress. When the pain did not stop, she started thinking that it was due to the stress she had at work. The fact that her father had died tragically from a terminal illness also was a factor.

No doubt many readers will find similarities between their own situation and A.'s Stress is a constant factor in all our lives. Most of us have quite intense lives and we may think we are dealing with it successfully. However, at this point it is important to note that one does not "get used" to stress. In the end, it affects us all, depletes our cognitive reserves, damages our mental state, and most probably affects us physically as well.

Sometimes, when we experience a series of failures (failure is subjective) or a sequence of problems in our personal lives, this is accompanied by a feeling of helplessness. All of us sometimes experience feelings like: "It's bigger than me," "I have no control over the situation," "Nothing I do helps."

It happens to all of us, but sometimes this feeling becomes a permanent pattern that accompanies us throughout our lives. We continue to think in this negative way when any new stressful situation comes along that requires us to cope. Psychologists call this "learned helplessness."

In a state of learned helplessness, we tend to passively accept the situation as it is (with responses such as, "That's life, what can you do?"). In such a situation we do not even try to change, and believe that things will happen regardless of whatever we do.

At this juncture, it is worth recalling Martin Seligman's famous study[9] conducted some fifty years ago. The study involved an experiment with two dogs. One dog was put in one cage and the other dog in another cage adjoined to the first cage. One of the dogs was administered an electric shock, but the shock was given based on the first dog's reactions and not its own actions.

That is, the dog that received the penalty in the experiment had absolutely no control over receiving or not receiving the shock. Nether its behavior or reactions affected whether or not it got the shock. The study showed that the dogs receiving the punishment regardless of their actions exhibited signs of clinical depression that were characterized by apathy, inaction, and lack of appetite, persisting long after receiving the punishment.

The same will be true with humans. Often, we tend to explain some negative event by enumerating factors over which we have no control. The way we perceive negative situations will affect the way we choose to deal with them. If we repeat this passive behavior often enough, it will teach us to be helpless. There are many instances of this. For example, situations where children experience continuing failure in their school work, or adults who fail to overcome ongoing economic problems.

Stress is part of our lives. We will always have to face challenges and meet the expectations of others or our own. It's a question of intensity and balance. Some levels of stress can have a positive effect, but this is not always the case, so it's wise to exercise extreme caution. Stress can have negative effects, and while some are not severe, they can impair our quality of life and be harmful to our health and well-being.

In the next section, we will look at the effects of stress on our bodies and the inception of illnesses, as well as the relationship between stress and emotional suffering. (Emotional pain syndrome.)

Dr. John E. Sarno's emotional pain syndrome, as outlined in his book, *The Divided Mind: The epidemic of Mind body Disorders*[10], he asserts that more than six million Americans are classified as having a mysterious and challenging ailment called fibromyalgia. People with this malady have been treated by an army of specialists, but none can clearly define the causes of the illness. Millions of others suffer from heart-burn and are treated with a plethora of different medications that are highly profitable for the companies that manufacture them, but their beneficial effects are unclear.

Sarno calls this a genuine epidemic. He argues that psychosomatics is a mind-body disorder that manifests as an actual physical problem, but it originates in the world of subconscious emotions. Psychosomatic illnesses are imagined illnesses whose origins are unclear. Conventional physicians sometimes associate these complaints with some period when the patient experiences a sudden high level of stress, which causes pain or an actual illness.

According to Sarno, subconscious feelings must be taken into account in any diagnosis of a medical problem that is unclear, including skeletal, lower back, respiratory, allergy, cancer, and even autoimmune disease. The psychosomatic processes begin with the subconscious, that part of the brain that is less known, which was first explored and delineated by Sigmund Freud. Psychosomatic disorder results from an imbalance between the subconscious and conscious mind. This is one of the common causes of psychosomatic disorders.

Let me tell you a story that describes a psychosomatic disorder. D., the director of digital communications for a certain government agency, told me about the day he recalled when he was driving his car and thinking to himself, "How long can this go on?"

Completely discouraged and almost devoid of energy, he decided at that moment he would not give in. Two years earlier, he had begun to suffer from an irritating and troublesome little cough that wouldn't stop. It grew harder and harder for him to speak at certain times, as almost every sentence took a great deal of energy for him to complete.

Running back and forth between specialists drained his finances and his energy. The physicians diagnosed him with a case of post-nasal drip, but no treatment was effective. D. was in a state of despair and this stress further worsened the physical suffering. The more he suffered, the more severe the symptoms became, and the worse the physical discomfort. He felt his doctors had no patience for people like him, who suffer from something that was not life-threatening, but still causes continual suffering and impairs the quality of life.

D. persevered, living his life as the model husband, the excellent father, and especially the successful executive. But this need to behave as if everything was normal, while nothing was normal, only increased the physical and mental price he had to pay. He began to suffer from symptoms of heartburn and esophageal discomfort, abdominal pain, blepharitis (an inflammation of the eyelids), and skin rashes.

D. came to the conclusion that he himself had to find relief from the physical and mental pain he was suffering with. One day, he came across an advertisement of a conventional doctor who had success treating patients with alternative medicine using the mind-body technique.

On the Internet, he found a video of this doctor telling his personal story. The doctor related that one day he couldn't walk or even get out of bed due to severe back pain. No treatment helped until he realized that although he was suffering from real physical pain, the source of the pain was not physical but mental. The very acknowledgment of this fact helped him begin a rapid healing process.

"What do I have to lose?" D. thought to himself. He contacted the doctor and told him his story on the phone.

The doctor listened and said, "I have good news for you. You are going to get better and you are going to do it by yourself. The source of all the physical suffering you are experiencing is mental. Once we understand the source of the tension, the physical problems will disappear and you will recover."

D. was skeptical, but thought, "I've tried everything else, it wouldn't hurt if I gave this a chance."

The doctor gave D. some simple mental exercises as well as using a homeopathic remedy to aid the mental process. After a few weeks, D. felt considerable relief. The symptoms had diminished and so the periods of relaxation between the various seizures increased. Over time, D. adopted a lifestyle that suited him and his health improved.

In many cases, the brain makes decisions based on automatic patterns, which we not only have no control over, but we are also unaware of. Take, for example, the emotion we feel in a situation where we are excited. Who among us would not be happy to control this excitement? Or take the blushing phenomenon. Blushing occurs when we are embarrassed or excited, without even wanting it. If we had control over it, we would have been able to prevent the blushing. And what about butterflies in the stomach? Can it be controlled and can we decide to feel butterflies in the stomach at a certain moment?

These phenomena are harmless and most of the time they are transient and that is why we don't give them much thought. If we are not aware that these phenomena are related to brain activity, we may suffer physically and think that this is a medical problem. Not only does the brain create a feeling or a semblance of pain, but an actual medical and physical problem.

In the case of D., every ophthalmologist noticed the dryness, every dermatologist diagnosed the rash, and every ENT specialist diagnosed the runny nose that trickled down his throat and interfered with his breathing, but none of them really understood what was causing these symptoms.

To explain such phenomena, one must understand that the brain produces bodily symptoms that originate with peptides in the autonomic nervous system[10].

A "peptide" in biochemistry is a compound made up of two or more amino acids. The peptides are molecules that participate in an internal brain-to-body communication system and play a pivotal role in these processes.

The autonomic nervous system is part of the peripheral nervous system and is responsible for regulating unconsciously directed actions, that is, actions not under the control of consciousness and behavior even when a person is asleep or unconscious, such as a regular heartbeat, breathing, secretion of sweat and saliva glands. This system is active twenty-four hours a day and as stated, is outside our cognizant system.

Our brain needs energy. It is vital and essential for its activities. The brain needs to manage this energy astutely and that is why some brain processes are autonomous. There are also many patterns of action that occur in our bodies, without our consciousness being involved.

Another interesting story is the case of "A."

A. is a close acquaintance of mine. He owns a small service company employing about twenty people. A. is considered a successful manager by any measure. From childhood, he grew up feeling like an outsider, one who had a strong need to please those around him: his family, friends, and employees.

A. works practically twenty-four hours a day to be considered a "good guy" by everyone. He is continually preoccupied with the question of whether those around him are receiving appropriate and satisfactory treatment, including his employees being content with the workplace he provides for them.

In his early forties, A. began to suffer from chronic headaches that no conventional treatment helped to reduce. He was prescribed various medications and also resorted to alternative healing methods, such as acupuncture, but nothing helped.

When I spoke to him about it, especially after he heard about my intention to write this book, he chose to tell me about the suffering he was experiencing that had adversely affected his quality of life.

I shared with A. my knowledge of emotional pain syndrome, knowledge I had gained not only from research, but also from my own personal experience. I explained to him the possibility that he may be experiencing an internal struggle that he is unaware of, because it does not exist in the conscious part of his mind.

We talked about there being a part of his personality that he very much wants others to know and appreciate, but also about the possibility that there is another part within him, a primitive component he is not aware of. I told him that in his subconscious, there was probably a fierce conflict raging with nowhere to vent itself. The expression of this subconscious inner struggle was the cause of his emotional, and subsequently physical pain.

What, then, is this primitive component of the brain? According to Freud, the personality is divided into three parts: the Id, the ego, and the superego.

- **The Id** – Is the primitive and unconscious part of the personality that is concerned with basic impulses. The Id is the impulsive (and unconscious) part of our psyche, which responds directly and immediately to basic urges, needs, and desires, regardless of the consequences or whether the act is responsible or even moral. This is the narcissistic part of man, the irresponsible and dependent part.

- **The Ego** – This part of the personality serves as an arbitrator in the conflict between the Id, the self who wants to do only what it wishes to, and the superego that wants to do what is right and responsible. The ego represents the physical and social reality and functions at the conscious level.

- **The Superego** – In the superego is where the ethical values of the individual, including the attitudes and moral perceptions that society has formulated, are stored. The superego is the conscience that develops as a result of a child's internalization of the prohibitions of his parents and other adults in regards to certain actions.

The Id is the part that does not want to please anyone or prove anything, even if it is the people closest to the person. If we look at it this way, we can say that A., who always wants his employees to be happy with him is actually subconsciously furious with them.

Perfectionism, or the striving for it, is one of the causes of unexplained illness and pain. A. in the present example, does not think of himself as a perfectionist, but his behavior and actions define him as one: hard working, responsible, achiever, striving to reach new goals, overcoming challenges, along with a sensitivity to the criticism of others as well as self-criticism. These all indicate a tendency toward perfectionism.

The desire to please others and win their approval, in addition to sacrificing one's own free time and personal needs, characterizes a perfectionist. These people are also disinclined to enter into a conflict and prefer compromise over confrontation. Arguably, the urge to be successful and perfect is, in fact, a subconscious response to a feeling of inferiority. The urge to be the best is equivalent to the basic and narcissistic urge expressed in the form of rage in the primitive part of the personality, the Id.

The psychological term "inferiority complex" describes the feeling within a person that he is inferior or of less value in some ways than others. Sometimes it is a subconscious feeling that motivates a person to overcompensate for it. In such a case, the person will work to achieve remarkable accomplishments or he will exhibit extreme antisocial behavior, or both. Unlike ordinary inferiority feelings that may act as an incentive for achievement, the inferiority complex is a lack of confidence that may manifest itself in avoidance of difficult situations in general.

In a study of one hundred four patients, it was found that the urge to be perfect characterized most of the subjects. For 31.5 percent it was the main cause of their illness, for another 36.5 percent the urge to be perfect was a factor in environmental pressure, and for 17 percent it was childhood abuse that pushed them to please those around them[10].

Another stress feature is called "daily stressors." This term usually refers to environmental stress factors that can be objectively observed: issues of work, family, career, finances, illnesses, concerns about aging, and mortality.

We often associate these issues with financial difficulties, or family disputes, but cognizance of our mental mechanisms allows for a deeper understanding.

Here are some examples: The need to be a perfect wife, a successful parent, or an exemplary child. All this creates pressure. The idea that only something external creates the stress is fundamentally incorrect. We are inundated with environmental and other stressors, but what they have in common is the existing gap or the tension between conscious awareness and the subconscious.

Most of us continue to mature with the years. It is part of our life's journey. At some point we will need to look after our aging parents. Lately, I have been dealing with a series of ailments of my eighty-year-old father. This is definitely a crisis situation, but it is important to understand that this is not a passing phase that will end when the parent's medical condition stabilizes. Our parents continue to age and become increasingly infirm, no matter how well we take care of them and how dedicated we are. Eventually, we all become vulnerable to the activity of the Id, the primitive mechanism that will respond with feelings of rage that are aroused within us.

The situation is even more extreme in societies where it is expected of offspring to care for their parents with the utmost dedication. This is a point worth dwelling on: the idea that the more devoted we are to our parents the less stress we will feel, does not stand the test of reality.

So, it is with "A," the devoted husband, father, and dedicated manager. A. expects his employees, his superiors, and the company shareholders to appreciate his efforts and that their appreciation should be reflected in material and other rewards. It is important to understand that dedication, no matter how boundless, is no guarantee that we will not feel stress or that stress will not be created.

The subconscious mind, that very same primitive survival mechanism, sometimes creates an opposite feeling to the existing sense of consciousness. My intention is to feel anger and a desire for change at the same moment. The tension between these two sensations, one that we are not consciously aware of, that produces in us a feeling of distress that will remain for a long time. This can be avoided if the person is aware of the conflict and tension and acts to change his thinking patterns, and even his lifestyle.

Assuming that a person's job is the major cause of the stress, there are some professionals (or friends) who recommend a change of occupation. I have read numerous articles describing radical changes senior executives have made in their careers. Some have become writers or lecturers, others have become tour guides or yoga instructors.

The gist of my message is that even if you choose to change your occupation – and there is nothing wrong with doing that – you have to understand that this is an external change, which is sometimes needed, but not necessarily for the stated reasons.

The deeper understanding that change begins within us, is awareness of what John Sarno calls the "divided mind"[10]. This is only the beginning of the solution. Our occupation does not necessarily have a direct relation to the level of stress we experience. Most of us are not aware of the fear that sometimes arises in our subconscious, a fear that also nourishes and intensifies physical suffering, illness, and symptoms of physical pain.

Many of the physical symptoms we experience are due to the same gap between the conscious and the unconscious, which transforms into anger in the primitive part of the brain and creates a feeling of stress. Freud postulated that the onset of symptoms was, in fact, subconscious self-punishment, and if the symptoms are not adequately addressed, a momentary resolution of one symptom would be immediately replaced by another symptom[10].

Sarno[10] argues that distraction serves as a mechanism to protect us from dangerous feelings, so when one symptom is replaced by another, the recognition it needs is guaranteed. This is a process that feeds on itself and as I emphasized previously, a physical change, such as changing jobs, would not necessarily resolve the underlying stress. Our brain will continue in the same routine, creating other symptoms to sustain the mechanism of maintaining consciousness. In fact, we are all two different people: Dr. Jekyll and Mr. Hyde.

Let's take another example. "J." is a brilliant, successful, high-level executive. He is a man who radiates calm and is always in control. He can be counted on to perform well, even in extremely stressful situations. However, J. has been suffering from irritation for a long time. Outwardly, he functions successfully, but subconsciously he is creating internal tension between being a "perfect manager" and the burning anger in his unconscious.

In such a conflict, the brain produces a distraction that manifests itself in physical symptoms that J. suffers from. The mind produces a formulation, whereby physical suffering is inferior in intensity to mental suffering. J. is unaware of the subconscious tension he is experiencing and is focused on the external stressors he is dealing with very successfully.

The physical symptoms that he suffers are actually symptoms that serve the brain's defense mechanism to prevent emotions, such as anger and frustration, from penetrating into the conscious part of his personality. According to Sarno, two conditions must be met in order for J, to recover[10]:

1. He must understand that the source of his physical symptoms is subconscious.

2. He must fully acknowledge and accept the facts and processes that led to his physical condition.

An interesting question arises as to why the brain decides that the symptoms will be type 'X' and not another? There is an important principle here. People experience the symptoms they have learned to expect. Symptoms are programmed and conditioned responses of the brain, regardless of anything other than what the person expects to happen in his subconscious mind. It is very similar to an involuntary "tic," such as blinking, pulling on the ear lobe, or rubbing your leg.

I have mentioned before the term "conditioning." This concept was coined by Russian scientist Ivan Pavlov following a series of experiments he performed. According to his theory, as soon as a stimulus is created, such as a prolonged state of stress, a response will be based on an automatic, reflexive pattern. This is actually the brain learning process. Following the reappearance of a particular stimulus (in Pavlov's theory it is called "unconditioned stimulation"), the response is also repeated.

The reaction can be a negative emotional reaction such as anger, frustration, or rage that derives from a negative childhood event. It can be negative feelings that come from expectations that you have to be perfect, or it can be anger resulting from stressful life situations, feelings of guilt, shame, fear, insecurity, or vulnerability.

By obtaining appropriate knowledge and understanding of the source of emotional pain, one can change this cognitive conditioning that turns the suppressed rage in the subconscious into physical pain.

Through daily practice of principles I will elaborate on in the following chapters, the brain can be trained to avoid thoughts of pain. One can simply cause the brain not to pay attention. This can be done by focusing on the psychological basis of the pain. You have to tell yourself that this is a distraction created by your brain and that you can overcome it.

How can that be? After all, we don't really have the ability to influence our subconscious. There is not one explanation, but many. One of them that I have adopted is that the physical response is actually a repetitive type of tic. It is a trick of the brain and if we can discover the trick, its effect will disappear, just like when you discover how to perform a certain magic trick, it loses its effect.

I will explain this another way. Picture a dark house with a basement. If you avoid going down to the basement, your thoughts will make you afraid of what is down there: a serial killer, or a vicious dog, or anything else that is a repressed fear. But if you turn the light on and go down to the basement, you will see that apart from some old furniture there are no ghosts and demons, the fear will dissipate.

We have no control over our emotions, but we can practice and train ourselves to think and respond in a way that will not cause us physical suffering or other pain.

According to Sarno, recovery is incredibly simple:

First, a comprehensive medical examination should be conducted. If no clear cause of your suffering is found and yet you are still suffering, then it may be emotional pain syndrome. The very knowledge and understanding that the source of your physical disorder originates in the emotional world is an essential step toward recovery[10]. Understanding that pain or illness can be treated and that our experience of physical suffering is shared by many people throughout the world is a significant part of the healing process of emotional pain syndrome.

In summary, we can picture ourselves as a stretched guitar string, but we must sense when it is over-wound and we should release and let go. When you recognize that happening, pause for a moment and look upon the physical symptoms and pain not as a problem, but as a signal from the brain, you will understand that your brain is signaling you for help.

Through the technique of identifying the physical symptoms that come from emotional pain, and by focusing on the conversation with the brain out loud, we can deconstruct the unprocessed mental tension expressed in physical symptoms. In my own experience, I can say that cognitive change will lead to behavioral change.

We must view physical symptoms as very sensitive sensors that, in stressful states, detect our volatility and signal that something has gone wrong. As soon as we look at them this way, we will stop being afraid of the appearance of symptoms. Our very awareness and knowledge will reduce the effects of the symptoms over time until we are fully healed.

Worries, Worries…

"Anxiety weighs down the heart, but a kind word cheers it up." **(Proverbs, 12, verse 25)**

Anxiety, or worry is defined as a state of mind in which there is a fear of what may come. Usually a worry is accompanied by a sense of stress involving feelings of grief, disappointment, anger, and apprehension. Indeed, every day, life provides us with a lot of concern: "Is my power point presentation good enough?" , "Am I prepared for the meeting?" , "How am I going to make my mortgage and loan payments?", "Will my son get along in kindergarten?"

An acquaintance reported to me that she could not sleep

for a whole week because her much loved and successful son had broken up with his girlfriend. The breakup was accompanied by her son's heartbreak. She so identified with his pain that she felt as if her own heart was broken. Worry gnawed at her anguished soul, "What if he doesn't get over it? Is he strong enough to cope or will he choose not to and harm himself?", "Will he get over it, or will the pain cause him to avoid any intimate relationship in the future?"

Worry is an emotion like anger, sadness, or joy. It is an emotion that feeds on itself. That is, the concern usually not only occurs in our consciousness, but it also develops there. Oftentimes, the intensity and extent of the concern are incompatible with objective reality, if there is one at all.

Concerns lead to additional concerns, often producing a nearly uncontrollable loop of worry. This can affect our daily functioning and produce other feelings such as guilt, anger, and frustration, sometimes leading to fear and anxiety.

Everyday worries usually last for a short time, then morph into other worries, i.e., only the issue changes. Sometimes, a particular subject becomes an almost obsessive thought that plagues us. The feeling created is that it is this the most burning issue in our lives; no other issues matter except this one.

Not long ago I was at a conference and met a company manager who I had a close friendship with. He looked forlorn and had a dreary expression on his face. I was interested in his well-being and he told me this, "Don't ask, there has been a drop in company profits and for several weeks now rumors have been floating around that cuts and layoffs are coming. I'm fifty, a longtime employee, and one of the ones who are the highest paid. I am positive I'll be fired at the first opportunity. I haven't slept since the rumors started. Nothing can reassure me, and my mind is full of terrible scenarios – getting laid off, problem finding another job, and a worsening of my financial situation. My wife is used to a high standard of living, and I'm afraid she won't be able to cope with the radical change. It will cause increasing tension in our relationship, lead to a breakup, and a cycle of ongoing suffering."

I looked at his gloomy face amazed, and answered him, "How have you managed to conjure all this up in your feverish mind? How and why did you decide that all this was going to happen?"

"I'm convinced of it," he repeated, shaking. "My wife won't be able to stand it, and she's the best thing in my life. It will ruin our relationship." – I won't continue belaboring you with the continuation of this long, depressing conversation.

Suffice it to say that a month later, I called him to see how he was doing. "Not great."

"What happened?"

"Don't ask. Management announced that the annual bonus will be cut by 30 percent and I've already made plans with my partner for a long family trip this summer. It really bothers me because we were really looking forward to it."

"And…is that all?" I asked in surprise.

"Yes," he said. "What do you mean? Isn't that enough?"

I pressed him and asked, "What about the *Sword of Damocles?* Were you ever in jeopardy of losing your job?"

"Ahh, that's over for now," he replied. "I was spared…this time around."

See how our consciousness works, or by another name "our tormented soul"? After all, a month ago this was a man whose very life was in the balance and saw himself collapsing financially. This was a man who imagined seeing his children only within the framework of a divorce settlement, who thought his life partner would leave him and find another, more successful man. He was washed up, a captive to fear, anxiety, and terror.

But even when it became clear to him that the scenario he had built up in his imagination would not come to pass, instead of freeing himself from worry and enjoying life and appreciating all the good things he had, he chose a new worry from the obsessive and disproportionate family of worries.

Annoyed and upset, I quickly ended the conversation and thought to myself how quickly we tend to shift from one worry to another. Is this a glitch in our brain's software? Are we programmed to constantly think the worst, and if it doesn't happen, do we automatically find ourselves something else to worry about?

I thought to myself how easily, most of the time, although irrelevant to our normal lives, we latch on to and exaggerate the consequences in the daily news headlines: "Iran Arms a New Bomb," "Crisis between Iran and the US escalates," "North Korea threatens stability in the region," "Serial Murderer Loose in Manhattan," and so on.

Not a day goes by that we are not bombarded with new concerns that are blown all out of proportion to our daily lives.

Religions also address the issue of worry. Both Judaism and Buddhism hold that everything is controlled by our way of thinking. Our consciousness produces worry, but not the opposite, which is joy. I need to be glad that, in fact, everything is relatively all right, I am alive, and if I am, it means that there are many more and varied opportunities to create, make a living, and enjoy life.

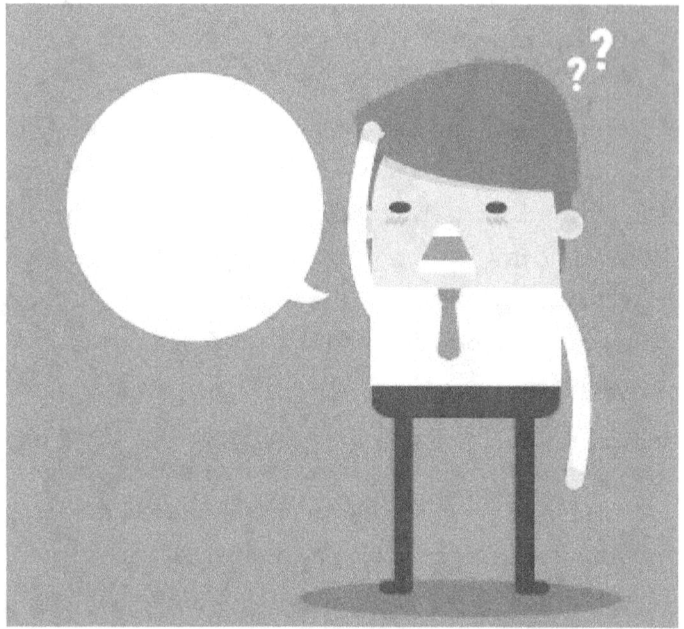

The frequency of joy apparently diminishes over the years. Look at your little children. Their lives are usually devoid of long-term worry. Why is this so? Because consciousness is still not well developed in them. Their parents have not yet instilled in them unnecessary anxieties or terrifying possibilities, bad memories, or unprocessed traumas.

The frequency of joy in our lives is so askew that it seems illogical to us that everything is actually all right. And overall, it really is.

The message for both the religious and the secular among us is clear. The way you see your life and what happens in it shapes our conception of our lives. On this subject, I want to be the bearer of good tidings: There is a remedy for worries, and not only by changing our awareness of a particular situation, but also by the adoption of rules to retrain our way of thinking in general:

1. Normalizing Emotions – In Buddhism, it is customary to state that if there is a problem and it has a solution, then why worry? And conversely, if there is a problem and it has no solution…then why worry? The message is that worry has no operative role and is only a warning sensor of potentially dangerous situations. To return the sensors to normal, you can use several tools:

A. Perspective – Think of yourself as part of something bigger. Every person is a private entity, but also a part of some larger group, organization, state, and society. Everyone is coping, not just you.

The difference between humans is not in the power and scope of their problems, but in their level of resilience to deal with them. At the end of the day everyone has worries, the proportions and perspectives make the difference.

B. Proportion – "It's not that bad." Try to look at a troubling situation from a different angle and contemplate what you can learn from it. It can be an opportunity for change and perhaps for improvement. In most cases, it is not an existential crisis, but only a crisis that is perceived as existential – and there is a profound difference.

C. Alternative – Look for ways to change the existing situation. There are always different options and in most cases change can be achieved.

D. Faith – It is important to believe that there is a solution and that any crisis can be resolved. Sometimes the solution requires multiple and various resources but they are certainly attainable.

2. Processing the Emotions – It is useful and desirable to summarize your day on a daily basis and note what the concerns were that accompanied it. Why were you worried? What caused them? How powerfully did we experience the feeling of worry? Is it repeating itself or is it a new feeling? Was there really a need to worry?

We will often find that our worries were for nothing.

3. Venting Emotions – It is useful and desirable to share your concerns with colleagues, friends and family. Merely sharing and describing your concern out loud, including the explanation of your reasons for concern, will immediately reduce its intensity. Worrying generally does not have an objective measurement, it is a subjective feeling. The power of worry depends largely on its mental processing. Venting emotion through sharing will undoubtedly help you to see things in proportion.

4. A Balanced Lifestyle and Daily Routine – Even when worries play a large part in your life, you must set and maintain a daily routine. The routine will make worrying only a minor part of your day. Appropriate nutrition and exercise are also vital. Exercise allows you to concentrate on the movements and causes a release from consciousness, even if momentarily, from negative thoughts and worries.

5. Manage the Crisis and do not let the Crisis Manage you – even if it is a crisis that is objective and the concern is real, the situation can be addressed. We would do well to define a crisis as an opportunity to change our way of life and improve how we behave or think. Instead of dwelling on the crisis and its possible consequences and results, it would be better to think about alternative solutions.

Focusing on the thought and energy in planning and then on the implementation will be very helpful. Identifying the sources of the crisis and recruiting a team of advisers to help prepare a crisis management plan will help you understand that the crisis can be managed and even "overcome." There is always a solution. Sometimes different resources such as time and money will be necessary, but there is always a solution.

6. Professional Tools – If necessary, professional advice is possible and necessary. Counseling can be specific to content, but it can also be on the overall cognitive level as well. Sometimes we are lost in a fog of thoughts that makes it hard for us to see the light. Professional counseling (mentoring, psychotherapy, and other therapeutic methods) can definitely help.

Fear, Anxiety, and Paranoia

Anxiety is seen as a negative, diagnosed phenomenon, but it turns out that as long as anxiety is monitored, controlled, and at low levels, it is actually beneficial and necessary for everyone, and certainly for career-driven professionals.

Based on my own personal experience, I believe managers need a certain amount of anxiety. Anxiety prevents the manager from becoming overly complacent, not to rely solely on his intuition, and to actually test everything.

As with any area of life, it is also important to be alert to the extent and balance of anxiety. Anxiety can take over the person and cause continuous restlessness. It bounces around in the depths of his consciousness and gives no relief, even in seemingly peaceful moments – in bed, on vacation, or even in the most intimate moments of life.

The Difference Between Fear and Anxiety

We often confuse fear and anxiety. Fear is a vital response for humans, much like for other animals. Fear is a defense mechanism designed to help us survive. It stems from a threat that can be identified at a given moment and situation. For example, a dog growling at us, a vehicle bearing down on us, loud shouting and threatening hand movements, terrorist attacks, and more.

When we deal with the fear of threat, it is both physical and emotional. In contrast, when we deal with anxiety, the specific threat is not really clear. When we are anxious about an airplane flight, it is not usually about the possibility of crashing, heaven forbid, but it is a complex result of information processed by the brain that classifies the situation as a subjective threat. This is my personal interpretation only.

In a state of fear, the feeling usually disappears as soon as the threat is removed. For example, if we reach a zebra crossing and a car approaches rapidly and honks, and we panic and respond appropriately, the fear will subside. But if we avoid crosswalks, swimming in the sea, or flying in airplanes, this is already a case of anxiety.

Anxiety has wide-ranging effects and time, and is usually expressed in three dimensions: the physiological dimension (accelerated pulse rate, momentary faintness, and pain), the behavioral dimension (avoiding the source that we believe created the threat or identifying it as a threat), and the psychological dimension (what is happening to me? Will it happen to me again?).

If we understand the differences between fear, anxiety, and stress, we can resolve some of the difficulties. Fear, as stated, is an evolutionary mechanism in face of a tangible threat; Anxiety is more difficult to deal with because it does not come from a specific event, and stress comes from a combination of components.

Of course, chronic stress can also be accompanied by anxiety or anxiety disorder. It is important to remember that today there are very effective treatment methods for all types of anxiety. There are also many techniques to deal with stress and regulate its effects. I will describe several methods in the book, and as was stated, a solution can be found for any situation.

The Difference Between Anxiety and Anxiety Disorder

Anxiety disorder belongs to a group of mental maladies whose sufferers experience intense feelings of fear. Anxiety disorder interferes with the proper management of one's life, and those who have it report real damage to their quality of life. Anxiety disorder causes those who suffer from it to avoid what they perceive as creating the anxiety.

Anxiety attacks are usually brief, but very significant in intensity. An attack is often accompanied by a sense of dread and panic, in addition to physical symptoms such as an increase in heart rate, tremors in the body, a tightness in the chest, a lump in the throat, as well as behavioral components that simulate paralysis and immobility.

Anxiety disorder is actually a mental illness. It is relatively new in its diagnosis as a disease yet is the most common of categorized mental illnesses. It is estimated that today at least 5 percent of the population suffer from anxiety disorder of varying intensity.

On the other hand, more and more voices are being heard, concerned about over-diagnosis of anxiety disorder. The common claim is that giving a prescription for drugs is too often and too easily done. Pharmaceutical companies have a financial interest in diagnosing anxiety disorder and establishing prescription drugs as the safest path to happiness, or in this case, to an anxiety-free life.[11]

It is important not to confuse feelings of stress and sadness, which in most cases are normal, with anxiety disorder which is a true neurotic disorder. You must understand that it is definitely possible to deal with feelings of anxiety, stress, and sadness, and that there are many different ways to deal with them effectively.

Dr. Ian Robertson is a writer, clinical psychologist, and neuroscientist. In his book, *The Stress Test: How Pressure Can Make You Stronger and Sharper,*[12] offers an approach that sees stress as a positive element. Robertson describes a long list of studies he and others have conducted on the relationship between the human brain, human behavior, and typical brain diseases such as Alzheimer's.

The book focuses on asking questions such as why do people react differently to the same stimulus? For example, failure on a test causes some of us stress and for others it is the beginning of a change and empowerment process. Robertson argues that stress at a given time and dosage can be a positive factor.

This is the paradox inherent in the phenomenon called stress. The stress appears when we are pushed a little beyond our appropriate arousal level. The level of arousal is the response of the autonomic nervous system to environmental stimuli or sensations.

The level of mental arousal is determined by the brainstem. When certain stimuli rise to a higher level than we are used to, the body feels it and the sensations are reflected in an increase in heart rate, an increase in blood pressure, an increased secretion of sweat, and increased muscle tension. Additional reactions can include increased urine output, a change in voice, and a change in the amount of oxygen consumed.

One of the famous models that describes the relationship between the excitation level and motor performance is called the "Reverse HS Model" or the "Yerkes-Dodson Law."[13] The law that these researchers outlined about one hundred ten years ago stated that when the excitation level is too high or low, the sensory information will not function properly.

If the excitation levels are too low, no sensory information will reach its target, and if they are too high, too much information will be available and will prevent the person from responding selectively to the stimulus. Each activity has a different optimization point on the excitation axis, and there are also interpersonal differences in response and excitation levels among different people.

The optimal level of excitation varies depending on the type of activity or the challenge. When we reach our optimum level, we will see an improvement in performance, but above our optimal excitation level we will be less successful. This situation occurs mainly in more complex operations requiring a high level of coordination and concentration.

When the level of excitation is high (say before an important test or game) or too low (say while watching television), this has an impact on mental and physiological processes. In a situation where the excitation level is low, one might expect low performance. For example, the inability to lecture to a crowd or a sense of blankness and paralysis during a test.

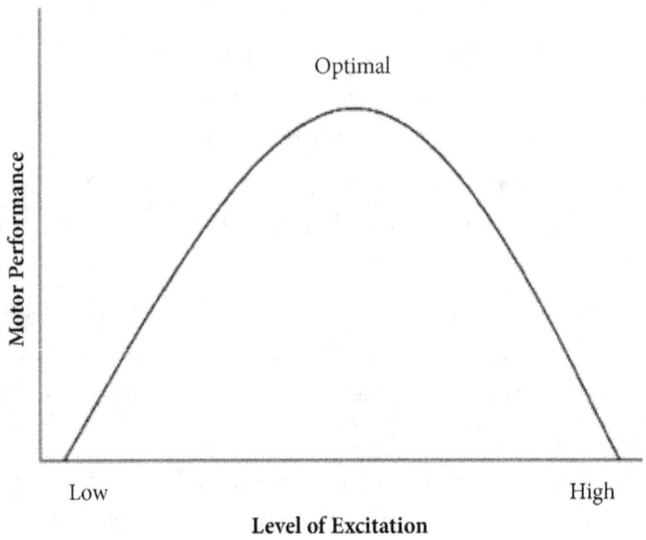

In his book, Robertson confirms the conclusions of the "Yerkes-Dodson law." In the famous experiment of 1908, mice were subjected to varying physiological pressure (using electric shock). Their conclusion was that exposure to moderate (versus high or low) stress would produce optimal functioning and performance.[13]

In studies conducted by Robertson, he came to a similar conclusion. As we push beyond our optimal excitation levels, the levels of noradrenaline become very high and flood the brain and body. The effect is positive but going beyond that will result in performance impairment.

Therefore, Robertson defines stress as a situation where the demands placed on us exceed our confidence in our ability to cope. In this situation people experience stress. The duration varies from person to person and depends on the circumstances. The stress usually lasts for a short time, but it can also take a long time. In this situation it becomes chronic stress.

In chronic stress states, cognitive function and memory are impaired and the risk of dementia also increases. Stress impairs and weakens our cognitive ability. However, Robertson claims that there is also positive stress. According to Robertson, what makes an event either an empowering challenge or a threat to us is the feeling of control.

People who believe that they have control over their lives, no matter what the objective reality is, will see stress as a challenge to be faces and not a frightening threat. His conclusion is that a positive attitude or as he calls it "reassessing the difficulty," allows a sense of control over the event and can reduce a person's stress levels.

As we saw in the previous chapter, when experiencing a difficulty or stressful event it is advisable to re-evaluate the difficulty by studying the factors that caused it. This is how we transfer the "management" of the incident from the amygdala (the security officer with the very sensitive alarm system) to the cortex (the conscious and thoughtful CEO) and we can consciously process the threat experience.

It is also worth checking out the emotional assessment that is connected with the event we experienced. These actions will help us to take away our sense of responsibility for being in this difficult situation. This in itself will allow us to have a certain sense of control over our lives and especially our emotions.

For example, if you are very pressured by important upcoming meetings, you can classify these meetings from now on as being important and interesting meetings that you are excited about. Classifying the event as exciting rather than stressful will reduce the immediate sense of anxiety. In the long run, this type of classification will train the brain to adopt patterns akin to excitement rather than stress.

In stressful situations, especially in prolonged ones and in times of crisis, the tendency is to see the difficulty as uncontrollable, as a situation in which your destiny is no longer in your hands. People who have been seriously ill or have suffered a severe loss describe this feeling well. I strongly believe that in any situation, however difficult, we still have some level of control.

Rona Ramon, the widow of astronaut Ilan Ramon, who was killed in the "Challenger" explosion, has been an impressive figure and a source of inspiration for many, recently passed away. In one of her interviews, she said she had asked her children to no longer engage in the questions of "Why?", "Why did this happen to us?", "Why now?", "Why did I deserve it?" She asked them to stop dwelling on the past and what went wrong, which allowed them to gain control of their lives.

The big mistake would be to think that stress is outside of us and that we have no control over it. Once we believe that, we will begin to fear and that fear will be our enemy. Later, we will be afraid of the fear itself. It will become the kindling to feed the fear and turn it into a severe case of anxiety.

In Scott Stossel's new book, *My Age of Anxiety*[14], he explains that through the development of mental resilience, anxiety can be controlled. At the opening of Chapter 12 of his book, he lists an important quote from a book called, *The Meaning of Anxiety*, written in 1950 by Rollo May:

"Anxiety cannot be prevented, but it can be reduced. The problem of dealing with anxiety is reducing it to normal levels, and then utilizing it as a stimulus to increase one's awareness, alertness, and one's zest for life." (Page 334)

Mental resilience can reduce the level of anxiety. A person's mental resilience is perceived as something genetic, a trait, or a characteristic that humans are born with. There is certainly a connection between genetics and traits such as resilience, but we often consider ourselves to be lower in resilience than we actually are.

Let's focus a moment on anxiety in the business world. Collins and Hansen have authored many books dealing with successful companies. They looked at what characterizes them.

One of their most successful books is, *Great by Choice: Uncertainty, Chaos, and Luck--Why Some Thrive Despite Them All.*[15] In this book, Collins and Hansen analyze companies that they call visionary companies, as well as shattering some of the myths in the management world such as "it takes a big idea to start a big company" or "visionary companies need charismatic and visionary leaders." Here is an example of one of the myths they shatter:

Myth – Successful leaders in a turbulent world are bold, risk-seeking visionaries. **Contrary findings**: The best leaders...observed what worked, figured out why it worked, and built upon proven foundations... They were more disciplined, more empirical, and more paranoid. (Page 9)

Collins and Hansen thus argue that the myth that visionary companies need charismatic leaders is wrong and should be shattered. According to their theory, the leaders of successful companies were laid-back and alert, and even paranoid. They were wary of the day when business realities would blow up in their faces and change.

Anxiety, therefore, characterizes many people, among them managers and executives. Anxiety is usually seen as negative due to its devastating implications. When anxiety is excessive (for example, disproportionate thoughts on the future), it can paralyze and, in particular, cause the manager to avoid acts or actions related to the source of the anxiety. In this context, a manager suffering from excessive anxiety will suppress progress and not facilitate it.

Another study conducted by Professor Tsachi Ein Dor and associates[16], found that anxiety also has adaptive sides. In a study they conducted among forty-six groups, they gradually filled a room with smoke as a result of a faulty computer. Participants in the study who were classified as emotionally anxious were quicker to identify the threat and the danger, and the group was able to function more effectively and respond appropriately to the threatening situation to which they were exposed.

Similarly, participants who had a tendency to avoid emotional confrontation responded quickly and fled the room, contributing to increased group confidence. The researchers concluded that the more anxious and avoidant members of the group are actually very important to the group, although they have difficulties adapting to a variety of situations in a social, emotional, or behavioral context.

Excessive anxiety is associated with decision-making processes in several ways. Anxiety has a deterministic effect on decision makers by influencing the way information is processed. Information processing in those with excessive anxiety is usually slight and simplistic.

In some situations, excessive anxiety can create a tendency to take extreme risks. It also usually causes attention to be diverted from the problem itself, as the attention is entirely on reducing the anxiety and controlling it instead of dealing with the problem[17].

The question is, "What is the right dose of anxiety?" There is no definitive answer, but it can certainly be argued that the optimal dose depends on the personality of the manager and the work environment. Dosage will be determined by trial and error. When a manager feels that anxiety is not reality-based, in other words, it begins to take control of his life and prevents him from performing essential actions, then he must stop and reassess.

The degree of real anxiety is what makes it effective and that is the key word. Effectiveness will help the manager to achieve realistic goals, to operate within a framework of uncertainty, to face difficulties, and most importantly, to make necessary changes.

Gathering ongoing information on market trends and an in-depth knowledge of the employees and their difficulties will help the manager handle the expected changes. Designing response-action scenarios can also help maneuver through difficult periods.

One of the important issues in making anxiety effective and not a paralyzing factor is simply the awareness of it, its causes, its consequences, and its ramifications. Suppose that one of the causes of anxiety for a particular manager from the pressure exerted by the company owners to increase profits, mainly by controlling expenses. Quarter-by-quarter, he manages to meet the goals. But there may be a gnawing fear of what will happen should he fall short in the next quarter? Competition becomes increasingly aggressive and he will have a hard time reinventing himself over and over.

And so it goes, "Soon I'll be fifty and if I don't meet my goals, I'll be laid off and find myself unemployed. I am accustomed to a high standard of living and there are few opportunities for reintegrating." These thoughts gnaw at the manager's feeling of security and are a cause for his worry.

How do we use this anxiety to make it effective and not paralyzing? First, live in the moment. Of course, it's also important to raise awareness, but you need to know that the prospect of success in the next quarter exists and is strong. And if it exists, then that is where it is worth focusing your energy.

When anxiety is controlled, it can allow you, as a manager, to come up with new ideas and reduce your complacency as well as that of your employees.

As a manager, it is important that you get to know yourself and identify what is causing you anxiety. Traumatic events in your past are definitely a factor. Assume that as a manager, you have been fired in the past due to poor performance. This trauma will be engraved in your memory and affect the degree of anxiety in your new workplace.

I have spoken to many executives who claimed that they had learned to be more cautious. Trauma and past memories have created a thinking pattern that can prevent them from taking action due to the fear of being hurt. For example, avoiding new close relationships and not sharing information with colleagues, or worrying about being too close to a superior to reduce the chance of getting hurt.

Studies show that experiencing the right emotion (anxiety, sadness, or happiness) at the optimal degree of frequency and intensity, and in the right context or situation, will enhance the capabilities of organisms[18] especially for persons of high intelligence.

Canadian researcher Penney and colleagues[18] investigated the relationship between intelligence and emotional disorders. They asked whether a thoughtful and caring mind was also a more intelligent mind. One of their conclusions was that there was a connection between the level of verbal intelligence and emotional disturbances such as reflection and apprehension. That is, a person with high verbal intelligence will analyze past and present events in greater detail, leading to a higher intensity of rumination and apprehension.

Reflection is typical of many executives I have met, especially characterized by dwelling on thoughts of their past experiences, not necessarily positive ones, and particularly past crises. Assuredly, the mere reflection on crises, and sometimes traumatic experiences, causes a higher level of anxiety. However, this is also an advantage, as reflection arouses the brain and allows us to function more sharply and perhaps more intelligently.

Reflection is basically a subconscious method in which the brain cooperates with a negative mood. The thought itself is not the problem, but the combination of the reflection with the negative thought leads to attention on the self. Usually it is characterized by self-reflection and focus on negative feelings, such as, "Why did this happen to me?", "I will fail," "All the bad things happen to me." And so forth.[19]

So, how do we manage anxiety? How can we make it possible for it to become an effective tool for living? First of all, awareness. The awareness that we allow ourselves a degree of anxiety will enable us to control it and make anxiety realistic and effective. Second, if we are managers, try to identify the factors that may increase your anxiety level. Divide them into groups: clients, colleagues, senior executives, shareholders, and consultants, including accountants, legal counsel, and business partners (suppliers, regulators, and others).

After dividing the factors into groups, we will try to map in each group who are the specific people who may be the main source of our anxiety. At the same time, match the person with a subject. For example, David works in my department and decides to quit his job.

Perhaps his departure is due to the dissatisfaction he experienced in my managing capabilities? Anxiety over this will happen next: "Will management see this as my failure as a manager?", "How will I do without him? After all, he has the knowledge and skills I need in my department."

Once we have mapped the groups, people, and subjects, we will try to refine the factors that are not necessarily related to one of the groups, such as deadlines, multitasking, heavy workload, emotional stress, the gap between available resources and expected results, high expectations, the gap between how I see the goals and how senior management sees them, conflict between family and work, a conflict between my investment in my work and the remuneration for it, etc.

We will now try to rank the factors according to their influence. Focus on what you see as the five key factors. Rate them by the way they affect you. How much do they really bother you, and how much do you regularly interact with them?

Mapping is essential. Already in the mapping process the intensity of emotions may be reduced as things will suddenly be seen in proper proportion. You might suddenly think, "What are we pushing ourselves for?" You might realize that almost every issue has a solution or a way to minimize its negative impact.

At this point it is helpful to include colleagues or other managers in the process. Interaction with others contributes to the control of the anxiety level.

For example, a major customer represented by a manager on his behalf, often complains about the level of service. Analyze the complaints and try to figure out what motivates him. Is it possible to find a solution? If you consult with colleagues you can formulate ideas for action and meet the complaints head-on. Usually this unmediated interaction will change how you feel. You might even find that this is a sympathetic man who, in your mind, has emerged as a frightening ogre. Change your approach. Not every complaint is a threat. See in such a situation an opportunity for improvement and customer retention.

In addition, to managing anxiety, try adopting a routine of moderate physical activity at the end of each day during which time you will perform one of the mapping-related issues. For example, during a moderate walk with a friend or spouse, tell them what happened during the day. Use a link to a specific group: "You know, today in a talk I had with my employee, she didn't stop crying and being resentful. She complained that I wasn't treating her properly. I thought it over and saw that I could give her a little more attention by having her meet with me every two weeks for a conversation. I will also assign her more challenging tasks."

During the conversation, try to define what emotion you are feeling. Usually, just having the conversation and defining the emotion will help the brain process the issue. Physical exercise will also help to release hormones that will make you feel more positive.

Another tool for mapping and reducing anxiety levels is the use of task priority techniques. The idea is to have clear schedules for task management. For example, allocate half an hour each morning for taking care of the most important tasks or at least plan how you are going to handle them.

It is also advisable to set expectations for each of the group members that we defined in the previous mapping. The process of setting expectations and afterwards coordinating expectations will reduce a feeling of frustration and the emphasis will shift from emotion to action.

Work at maintaining a positive relationship with your employees, especially your colleagues. A large-scale study of twenty-nine hundred managers by Norwegian group of researchers[20] revealed that managers who had a positive relationship with their employees were less affected by performance anxiety, which means that anxiety was controlled and not excessive.

They also reported that they had a positive and supportive relationship with their subordinates, who on their part placed great confidence and faith in their managers. This is because the relationship was built on trust and mutual commitment.

According to the above study, there are four factors that create an atmosphere of stress in the workplace: workload and deadlines, emotional stress, a gap between management's demands and realistic capabilities, and a gap between family and work expectations. Six out of ten Norwegian executives stated that they experienced too heavy a load resulting from rigid schedules and workload tasks and commitments.

Anxiety is certainly a significant factor in all our lives, and especially in the lives of managers and employees. To some extent, anxiety serves as a motivating factor for action, and even allows for more cautious and moderate decisions.

In organizations, and perhaps even in families, where it is possible to process and normalize emotions, the negative power of anxiety (a subjective measure) will be reduced.

Paranoia and Stress

Paranoia is usually linked with an extreme level of suspicion. The employees of an organization are part of a culture in which there is generally not much trust between its members at various levels. Building and establishing trust is a long, complex process.

Mutual suspicion is a given among employees as well as managers. It is characterized by the need to summarize company discussions in the form of "protocols," a need to formulate back and forth emails with the achieved understandings and, above all, to live with a constant sense of persecution, organizational but also personal persecution.[21]

In a clinical sense, paranoia is a disease whose sufferers see reality in a distorted way and who feel constant persecution and danger from those around them. These false ideas are part of their everyday life and make up the whole world of the sufferer.

It is important to note that paranoia also exists in people who are not labeled as mentally ill. These people experience a feeling of persecution at lower intensity and their lives are on the normative path. Executives in any organization should adopt this type of a sense of persecution, which emanates from a slight suspicion, minimal, and under control.

Andrew Grove, in his book, *Only the Paranoid Survive: How to Exploit the Crisis Points That Challenge Every Company*[21], believes in the value of paranoia. He argues that a manager should always be vigilant, and not only that, but he must also establish this approach in the people close to him.

It is also assumed that formal planning, as rigorous and methodical as it may be, is not able to predict all of the changes, and thereby intensifies their impact. It is important to plan, but not to the extent that we sacrifice flexibility, responsiveness, and maneuverability.

Grove not only imparts this message as managers in the organization, but also links it to our own career management. Especially in the current era, we must understand that even if we plan our careers in great detail, we must be ready to maneuver and change. We must be able to respond in real time, because in the world of employment we will all have to deal with personal and career challenges.

How does all this relate to our subject? A great deal. Anxiety, worry, paranoia, and fear are different in degree, but they are also quite similar. They exist in each of us; certainly, within the managers among us. We can use these feelings as tools to help us improve our management skills. With the right intensity, dose, and frequency, each of these feelings will make us better managers.

Here is another example. Recently, the business run by "J." is experiencing unexpected growth. This resulted in a significant increase in revenue, but the number of complaints and dissatisfaction of some of their customers increased. J. felt overwhelmed. He kept getting emails with complaints that were more and more aggressive, such as, "The response time at the call center makes no sense", "If you don't improve this situation, we will consider discontinuing doing business with you," and so on.

J. was frustrated. He was working as hard as he could, but every such email made him feel he was losing control. Negativity flooded him: "What will my top managers think about me?", "What will the board say if we have to report that a customer has left us because of poor service?"

Suddenly, all the positive things he did were diminished and he was only occupied with the negative thoughts. In such situations, a feeling of anxiety overtakes us. We feel tired, lack energy, or a desire to face reality. Then follow the line of thoughts, like, "I'm exhausted, tired out. I need to find another profession."

The thoughts keep hounding us: "Maybe I'll go back to be a college lecturer, or a consultant? Anything but what I'm doing today." These thoughts notwithstanding, however, we know we have to pull ourselves together. And we are still frustrated. While we do all that we can to find solutions, yet everyone is dissatisfied: even the hard-working employees feel unappreciated, as do the managers who are not getting the expected result.

At this moment, we must understand that there are situations over which we have limited control. We can continue to live our lives berating ourselves, with a growing sense of persecution and fear of the worst. But is the worst happening at this very moment? Probably not. And suppose things do get worse and we have to take responsibility, give back the keys to the office and go home. Is it the end of the world? Or could it simply be a strategic turning point in our career (SIP) as Andrew Grove called it?

From an evolutionary standpoint, our brain is habituated to think the worst, simply to allow us to survive. In modern life, this behavior of the brain is not always to our benefit, especially when these feelings get out of hand. You have to be aware that these are usually subjective feelings and are, therefore, also under our control.

Remember that we can do a great deal to keep stress from overwhelming us. The key principle is that the person has to take control of the situation, to train the brain to change thought patterns, and no less importantly to reflect, share, and process. Stress management strategies will reduce its intensity, regardless of what is going on around you.

Cognitive Load – a Case of Overload

I stood helpless in front of the receptionist at the health club where I work out. I was stressed, tense, with innumerable thoughts running through my head.

"Are you sure?" I asked her, in a slightly trembling voice. "No one brought them in?"

"Sorry," the young woman said sweetly.

"What am I going to do?" I said anxiously. "How am I going to get home without the car, and what do I tell the insurance company?" Horrible scenarios had begun to flood my brain. "Calm down!" I commanded myself, you only lost the keys to the car.

I decided to gather a group of the gym trainers and we searched every inch of the place but found nothing.

"Go up to the parking lot and see if the car is still there," one of them advised me.

I walked heavily to the elevators and exited fearfully to the parking lot where I was sure I had left my car. I walked all around it, but the car wasn't there.

I decided to go back to the club and try my luck again when I heard a voice behind me, "Here you are! I've been looking for you for half an hour. I have to close the car wash already. Your car was ready a long time ago."

I don't know what I felt at that moment. Relief that the car hadn't been stolen or embarrassed by what I would have to say to the trainers who helped me search for the keys. Maybe I'm starting to get symptoms of Alzheimer's…?

The above is an example of a common and typical case of "cognitive load," or "mental load." In cognitive psychology, this is defined as a mental effort that overloads our working memory while performing a complex task, such as decision-making or learning.

In 1988, John Sweller[22] developed the Cognitive Load Theory used by cognitive psychologists in various fields, but mainly in education and decision-making. This theory explains how, in our busy lives, we place a heavy burden on our working memory.

What exactly is this "working memory"? The term is borrowed from the world of computer science. Computer working memory is what allows the computer to perform its ongoing operations. The human brain's working memory contains all the information for active and current use to perform current tasks here and now. Working memory serves as a short-term processor and is part of our consciousness.

Suppose we attend a meeting and see a presentation that contains certain data. This information will be contained in our working memory and await the use we will make of it. Working memory is a processing space associated with a person's conscious mind, as opposed to long-term memory which is a repository of information stored for a long time.

Working memory not only allows us to calculate the bill at a restaurant or remember the data from the presentation, it mainly allows us to experience of being present in the moments, in the here and now. This moment is encoded in our memory visually, spatially, and aurally.

As employees, and particularly as managers, working memory is an essential component of both the decision-making and planning processes. Working memory allows memory to be recalled from previous experiences, optimizing the planning of future tasks. Working memory serves as a sophisticated router and filter. Information is absorbed, filtered, processed, and some of it goes into long-term storage.

Studies show that this process can take up to two minutes. Suppose you are at an important meeting. A properly working memory will allow you to split your attention among the others present, gather information from everyone, filter it, and process it.

Obviously, you can't remember everything that happened at the meeting, you might just remember small parts of it. This has to do with the capacity of your working memory and the processing you have done. If at the end of the session, or even during the meeting, you summarize the important points or discuss your impressions with a colleague, a greater amount of information will be stored in your long-term memory.

What, then is the working memory capacity? Our capacity for sadness or joy (depending on your perception) is limited. It reaches its peak around adolescence and at its peak it contains up to seven information details, but equally important, it is also one of the reasons that it is sometimes hard for you to remember where you parked your vehicle.

If while you were looking for parking you were talking on the phone and thinking about your child's after school activity, you might not remember afterwards where you parked.

There are many theories on the subject, and opinions differ on the number of items you can efficiently store. Various techniques can help increase memory capacity. In my opinion this is a very individual matter and depends on many factors. It is advisable for each person to discover the limits of their daily working memory.

The conclusion is clear. Modern life is chock-full of information that comes to us from all directions, and it is all about a very small part of the brain that has its limits. The cognitive load, and often the emotional load, creates a mental load on us that is very difficult for us to cope with successfully.

So, what's the solution? How do we reduce the mental load in our lives?

The less packed our work memory is, the clearer our decision-making. Research shows that when we experience cognitive load and our working memory is full, the brain activates a mechanism of automatic responses. These responses are quick solutions, but they are not necessarily good ones.

This is easy to illustrate with the following story. I was returning home from a busy day and while I was still on the road, my partner called me, "Sweetie," she began.

You have no idea what I was feeling. A feeling of crisis and cold sweat. My many years of experience had probably taught my subconscious that the combination of my partner's voice with the term "sweetie" will be followed by a series orders and admonitions.

"Yes, dear," I replied.

"Dearrrr," she went on, making things sound worse. "Remember I asked you to buy tomatoes at the supermarket?" And immediately, without waiting for my response she added, "You forgot, as usual. So, before you come home make sure you finish the rest of the shopping. Oh, and we're out of milk, tea, and sugar, and by the way I sent you a few more things to buy on WhatsApp."

Tired, exhausted, and anxious, I had trouble processing this information in my very limited working memory. (By the way, in my opinion there is a significant difference between women and men in the utilization of working memory. Women have a much greater capacity.)

I drove to the supermarket and bemoaned my fate. All I wanted to end this day was a hot shower, dinner, and maybe a little slouching in front of a flickering screen called TV.

I sighed and got out of the car and walked toward the supermarket entrance. I took a cart (automatic operation) and started roaming around the aisles. Suddenly I stopped, "What did she ask me to get?"

I opened the SMS and saw a bunch of groceries, but I was sure she had asked me for more. I stood there, worried and lost for a full five minutes. I couldn't remember what she said to me to add to the list, and I really didn't want to call her, because that would end with a long sermon about how I never listen. In short, out went all thoughts of a pleasant evening ahead.

Feeling downtrodden, I shuffled idly by the shelves and the thought came to my mind, why not buy almost everything I could. Better to get a reprimand for too much than to return without the things you were asked to bring. After a full hour, dripping with sweat and an accelerated heartbeat, I showed up on my doorstep carrying several heavy shopping bags.

"Honey," I began, apologetically. "I'm really sorry."

My wife looked at me with wide eyes and asked in a panic, "What's the matter?"

"No, no, it's nothing. It's just there was a sale on at the supermarket. Buy two items and get the third for free, so I thought you'd be glad if I bought out about half the store…" I was pleased with the story I had made up, but my partner was not impressed.

"Third item free, huh? Sure, sure, again you forgot what I asked you to buy!"

So, we now realize that in a state of mental strain, our physical resources are in short supply. One of the implications is that decision makers will shorten processes and respond to automated responses, meaning they will utilize their default choice. In addition, mental overload will impair our motivation to perform the tasks and have a deleterious effect on our performance.

It is also known that emotional stress, often created by depression and anxiety, will cause us to have a familiar feeling of mental weakness and emptiness. Some would describe this as "having no air," characterized by a lack of motivation and desire.

Pay attention to various signs. For example, do we tend to often forget routine tasks, even common things like taking time to have a meal during the work day? Do we wake up in the middle of the night or very early in the morning with inexplicable physical pain? Are troublesome thoughts incessantly bothering us? If you have experienced one or more of these symptoms, you were most probably in a state of mental overload. What to do?

There are several steps you can take to ease your cognitive load. Here are some examples:

- A short session of mindfulness or any other type of meditation will help to "empty the mind" and make room in your working memory. Practicing meditation will also reduce emotional clutter.

- It is desirable to reduce your amount of alternatives and reduce your choices, even in what to wear, or what to eat, but particularly cut down on the number of tasks required in a given amount of time.

- Documentation: I use a dedicated app to document my thoughts, ideas, and experiences. This allows me to process the points at a later time, not at the moment, but when it suits me best.

- Vigilance and a good mood are highly recommended. They help to improve the efficiency and capacity of your working memory and reduce cognitive load.

It is important to practice different ways of using your working memory. For example, trying to remember pictures rather than words, using your imagination for illustration or linking certain things to other things you know, and most importantly, being aware of the phenomenon and not being stressed, because like everything else in this life, it has a solution.

CHAPTER FOUR

COGNITIVE – PSYCHOLOGICAL ASPECTS AND STRESSORS

"Human happiness is less dependent on objective conditions and more on our own expectations."
(Yuval Noah Harari, 21 Lessons for the 21st Century)[1]

Assessment and Coping: Modes of Repression, Denial, Avoidance, Addiction, and Stress.

One of the common paradigms is that stress causes an increase in blood pressure. The argument is that if something stresses, upsets, or worries us, our blood pressure will rise. Also, if our lifestyle contains many such tensions then we will suffer permanent damage from high blood pressure.

This explanation is problematic. Usually when something stressful occurs, there is indeed an increase in blood pressure, but only for a very short time. While some people may suffer from chronic blood pressure fluctuations, for many of us the reason for these fluctuations is not necessarily due to poor nutrition or an unhealthy lifestyle.

If we put a blood pressure gauge on our upper arm, it seems perfectly normal that during the day we will have ups and downs in our blood pressure. Another explanation for high blood pressure is from the field of psychology.

The origin of the increase in blood pressure may be repressed emotions that we are not aware of and which emanate from the subconscious mind (as we have described in detail regarding emotional pain syndrome). In many cases, chronic diseases such as blood pressure difficulties originate from the suppression mechanism.

The suppression, or repression mechanism, allows us to move thoughts that are difficult for us to accept or cope with from the consciousness into the subconscious. Suppressed aspirations and thoughts continue to exist in the subconscious and may manifest in various symptoms.

If we lie on the clinical psychologist's couch, we may be undergoing psychoanalysis treatment. Psychoanalysis seeks to retrieve repressed material back into consciousness, so that it can be dissected and discussed rationally.

Repression is a mental defense mechanism that psychology refers to for the transfer of memories, feelings, impulses, or thoughts from the conscious to the subconscious due to their threat to the "self."

Repression allows to control strong impulses that other defense mechanisms cannot control. The repression is done on a one-off basis, but later on, there is a constant investment of mental energy required to maintain the content in its repressed state, as they continue to operate unconsciously.

A clue to the existence of repressed experiences, emotions, and thoughts can be found in dreams, slips of the tongue, and slips of the pen. It is important to note that although repression is an effective mechanism, it is also dangerous since the detachment of the "self" from whole parts of the person's life, emotions, and cravings can severely affect the well-being of the personality and be a source for engendering mental illness and limiting the perception of reality.

The brain usually represses events, people, and places that have negative emotional connotations. For example, a business or personal failure, or a result contrary to expectations, can be repressed because of their threat to the "self" and the person's self-image as a successful, fair, honest person and the like. Repression works alongside another psychological defense mechanism called "denial."

Denial is a cognitive mechanism to deal with negative emotions through the repression of the circumstances that caused them. In the case of denial, we subconsciously stop thinking about the issue or the situation. We believe that if we don't think about it we will not suffer the consequences of that particular situation.

For example, if I am constantly overdrawn at my bank, it is a cause for stress. If I reflect on it, I would most likely change my spending habits, but if I deny the situation, I will see it as the bank's problem, not mine. That way, I reject personal responsibility and if there is anything I really want to buy, I do so without fear.

Sometimes denial is actually a good option. If it is a short period of time, denial can be an effective coping mechanism for pain or stressful events. Suppose you recently suffered from painful indigestion. We can choose to say, "It's nothing, probably something I ate or it's from the antibiotics I took recently."

If we do not choose to use denial, we could begin to

think that these abdominal pains are a sign of cancer. These thoughts will cause us acute stress and set off a whole reactive chain. In a case like this, denial is recommended to enable us to continue to function normally. In most cases, the problem will go away by itself.

The thing is, that although this is a defense mechanism, the upshot of denial is usually negative for most of us. Denial creates a circle of negative feelings that can create resistance and a waste of energy.

In 1984, the psychologists Richard Lazarus and Susan Folkman published their book, *Stress, Appraisal, and Coping*[23]. Further to the studies done by Lazarus a decade earlier, they argued that not all of us are affected by stress in the same way and that the reason for the differences is the way we choose to cope.

Some of us will deal with stress by avoidance or attack, while others choose to deny and rationalize. The fact that most of us will be affected during our life cycle by stressful events is unavoidable. However, what is important, is the way we choose to cope with the stress.

Coping strategies are modes, mechanisms, and cognitive-based behaviors that we can all learn, adopt, and refine our skills in dealing with stressful situations.

Life is full of situations that can cause us stress, but it is our choice of how to interpret them. A negative interpretation and a tendency not to deal with the stress is the one that according to Lazarus and his associates causes negative stress. The focus should not be on an effort to reduce the stressors, but on how to adopt an effective coping strategy.

Stressful situations are all around us and it is important

to know how to deal with them. Our response to them is a product of interaction between man and his environment. This interaction is assessed continually, consciously and unconsciously. The way we cope depends on our interpretation of the situation that we experience. We may have to cope with a scarcity of resources (mental resilience, time, etc.).[24]

The two essential processes in this interaction are coping and appraisal. Appraisal refers to an ongoing process where we evaluate what is going on around us in relation to our personality, values, and beliefs. In situations where our brain receives signals of danger and emergency, we constantly ask ourselves (not necessarily consciously) two essential questions, "Am I okay? And what can I do?"

Situations that we consider to be important to us, but we have little control over, will be perceived as dangerous. Conversely, those situations that we consider to be important, over which we have strong control, are usually classified as challenging.[24] It is an emotionally demanding process and we may experience anger or sadness in the event of danger, or elation and enthusiasm in facing a challenge.

After labeling the situation using the stress appraisal, we will select the means of dealing with it. Selected ways of dealing with stress are a function of beliefs and thinking patterns. There are several ways to deal with stress: ignore the problem, look at it with humor, or get support from close friends and family. There are also other ways, such as avoidance or escape or even blaming external parties for our situation such as others around us or the environment.

Most of us choose strategies that have worked for us in the past, but we try to be open to new ways as well. New information, learning, and sharing are of great importance. Here are two other ways to deal with a specific problem:

- **Problem-Focused Coping** – deals with the problem by finding a solution, or the opposite: momentarily avoiding coping with the problem. For example, you were called in for a meeting to discuss your possible dismissal and loss of your job. A way of dealing with this stressful situation would be to try to think of other ways to make a living in the short term or, alternatively, to do nothing for the moment. An approach like that can actually be comforting: "In any case I have time. First, I'll go to the meeting, and see what happens, and then decide what to do."

- **Emotion-Focused Coping** – relieves the emotions associated with the stressful situation, even if the situation itself is unchangeable. For example, if someone is seriously ill and there is no solution or cure, they can try to adopt positive ways of thinking and maintain their morale because there is nothing they can do about the disease at the moment.

In summary, we can say that it is advisable to try to deal with problems through sharing and focusing on the problem or emotion. Although many people use repression or denial, these are not the most recommended ways, because by choosing them we will pay a heavy price, both emotional and functional.

The Stress Mindset

Stress does not just occur as a response to cognitive, physiological, or behavioral changes. Recent research in the field shows that everyone has their own perception of stress.

The perception can be positive, which means that stress has a positive effect and can be a catalyst for development in various areas of our lives such as in our careers. In this case, stress is considered to be inseparable from a successful, career-oriented, and ambitious lifestyle.

We cannot move forward in life without some pressure. However, where stress is seen as negative, we see it as harmful and having deleterious consequences for our lives, and so it is better to avoid it or at least reduce its intensity as much as possible.

One of the studies on this subject was conducted by Israeli researchers[25], who participated in an American and Israeli research group to identify how stress perception affects stress assessment. At the heart of the research was the argument that the way we experience the degree of stress is related to our individual pattern of thinking about stress.

Suppose I see stress as having a positive impact on my life and especially my work. It can happen that when one of my employees tells me that he is going through a particularly difficult, demanding, and disturbing period, I will nod my head but think to myself, "What does he want? A little stress is a good thing." How I, myself, see stress will affect how I perceive its effect on those around me.

Not long ago, a colleague told me that she had gotten an important promotion, but from that moment on she started experiencing severe anxiety. Disturbing questions flooded her mind, such as, "What do I need this for?", "How will I cope with the stress at home and at work, and how do I balance them?" Her stress manifested itself in severe physical and mental symptoms.

Because I was in the middle of writing this book, I felt a strong sense of empathy for her. I identified with her emotionally. The way I perceive pressure clearly affected my approach.

Conversely, if she had shared her feelings with her managers, they might have considered this a weakness. If we are aware that there are diverse ways of thinking, we can ask ourselves, "Have we projected our own perception of stress on the person telling us his story?"

Personality Traits and Stress

I am not an avid fan of classifications and patterns, but I have learned that sometimes these can help, especially when we talk about changes in behavior and stress.

There is a debate among researchers as to whether each person has inherent personality patterns that define his or her behavioral choices or whether our interaction with the environment is what influences our personality.

Let's take a look at a sales manager at an advertising company. In the past week he sent out several price quote bids to clients and got back many rejections. He may convince himself the first time this happens that there is always a next time, but when rejections occur in succession it can be perceived as failure.

The manager will be less calm and more prone to anger,

and even if he continues to project outwardly that all is well, he may be filled with doubt and frustration that his anticipated bonus might be fading away…

On the other hand, another manager might try harder to succeed. This manager could blame the financial situation, and not himself, for the rejections. He will gather his courage to find a solution and hope that in the long run, things will balance out.

In the late 1950s, a pair of researchers named Meyer Friedman and Ray H. Rosenman[26], identified two distinct personality types. The study, which went on for approximately nine years, involved a group sampling of male subjects.

Eventually, the researchers identified two types: type A, the ambitious type who is always under pressure and in a constant state of competition, and type B, a gentler, more relaxed and calm type personality.

If you identify with the first manager, you will be diagnosed as personality pattern type A, and if you choose the behavior of the second manager, you will be diagnosed with personality pattern type B.

The study found that the temperamental nature of type A increases their chances of suffering from stress. The main reason for this is that their nervous system is prone to hypersensitivity (hypertension, heart rate, and adrenaline) and their rate of reaching relaxation is slower.

In addition, in type B, the cholesterol level is lower relative to type A. Hypersensitivity in type A's neuronal system and its slower relaxation rate compared to type B (when stressed), leads to higher blood pressure and faster heart rate than type B.

The following is a summary of the characteristics of the A and B patterns:

Type A: People demonstrating competitive and goal-oriented behavior. They feel a sense of urgency, and it is hard for them to relax. They become impatient and angry when met with rejection. Although they are self-confident, they are, in fact, full of personal doubts, and push themselves to achieve as much as they can in the shortest time possible.

Type B: People who are able to relax without feelings of guilt and work without overdoing it. They don't feel pressured by time; they are patient, and slow to anger. Type B will be cautious and examine several action scenarios. Type B is seen as more conservative and less likely to take risks.

If you have identified yourself as having type A characteristics, don't panic and try to relax. Typical type A behavior can be changed through proper training and treatment.

In addition, healthy lifestyle awareness may reduce the physical impact of stressful conditions in type A. Among the desired activities are proper nutrition, exercise, avoiding smoking, drugs, and alcohol.

Obviously, life is more complex than categorizing each person as one particular type of personality. I think most of us have some dominant personality traits, but with life experience we have added traits from other personality types. This is why we can characterize ourselves as having a dominant personality pattern, say type A, with some of the characteristics of B.

Some people would define themselves as type as AB or A-. That is, a type that is still competitive and goal oriented and wants things done in his own way, but the shared characteristics of type B add balance and make this person calmer.

In contrast, types whose dominant personality pattern is B, but who also have personality characteristics of type A, will still be very task-oriented, but they will add a dimension of caution, paying attention to details, and being more conservative.

In recent years, studies have identified two other personality types, labeled C and D. Type C is characterized as a lecturer or repressor type. These are people who love details. They are not assertive and tend to neglect their own desires in order to please others.

This lack of assertiveness can cause depression or stress. The behavior is characterized by conformity and passivity to some extent. In organizations and families, they will be the ones who are designated as disciplined workers or obedient children.

The downside of this type of personality is that even if they are in distress, they will not seek help or access psychological treatment on their own initiative, so as not to hurt their image. Also, these are people who tend to repress feelings or have a tendency to experience all stress as negative. They are inclined to accept their fate as inevitable and can easily fall prey to despair and helplessness.

Type D people tend to suffer from clinical depression. This personality pattern has a propensity to look at everything that happens in a negative way. Usually, they will present themselves as suffering from negative emotions.

Type D is characterized more than others by feelings of depression, anxiety, anger, low self-esteem, and especially social isolation. They are constantly tense, and it is likely they will suffer from emotional eating. These types will experience stress situations as very negative especially because they do not have the tools to deal effectively with mental stress and they will suffer as a result.

Research on these personality patterns finds that these traits are reliable predictors of future heart problems, even more than medical and other traditional risk factors. The main reason for this is because of the way they perceive stress. When we react negatively to stress, biological processes occur in our bodies, but it is more than that.

Type D's tend not to seek help, they do not share their distress, and they drown their grief in eating, not exercising, smoking, and drinking alcohol to excess, which are all detrimental to their physical well-being.

The Five Factor Model (The Big Five) and Stress

The Five Factor Model or the Big Five was developed about thirty years ago by psychologists Paul Costa and Robert McCrae.[27] The model, which has remained one of the most important and prominent in the field of personality attributes, asserts that the causes of human behavior are linked to five key dimensions of human personality:

- Openness to experience (inventive/curious vs. consistent/cautious)

- Conscientiousness (efficient/organized vs. easy-going/careless)

- Extraversion (outgoing/energetic vs. solitary/reserved)

- Agreeableness (friendly/compassionate vs. challenging/detached)

- Neuroticism (sensitive/nervous vs. secure/confident)

According to this model, individual personality can be defined based on these five dimensions.[28] The model was developed by a statistical method of factor identification mathematically derived from a questionnaire distributed among surveyed samples and was based on experimental studies (this is one of the main criticisms of the model).

Critics claim that relying on analysis from questionnaires is problematic and raises questions about bias (because of the reliance on self-report).

The Five Dimensions Model

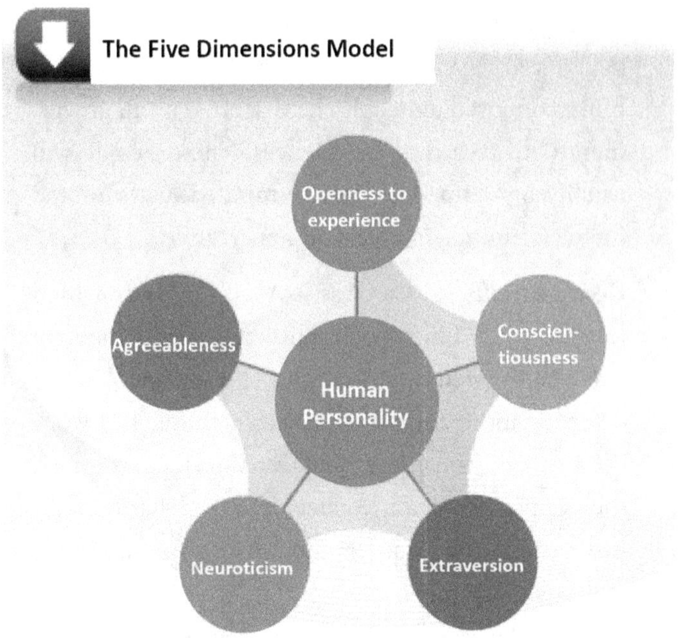

A basic assumption supporting this theory is that these traits stem from our biology, that is, we are born with these traits and as we develop and interact with the environment they grow and become stronger, eventually stabilizing around age thirty.

It is interesting to note that traits such as neurotic, extroverted, open to new experiences tend to diminish with age, while conscientiousness and compassion grow stronger in most of us over the years.[29]

An Outline of the Five Traits of Personality According to Costa and McCrae[30]:

- **O**pen vs. Wary – Those who are open to experiences have a well-developed, creative, and curious imagination as opposed to people characterized by an unwillingness to face new experiences. These people will usually be defined as narrow-minded, with limited interests, unimaginative, and noncreative.

- **C**onscientious vs. Careless – A person with a high level in this dimension indicates a willingness to work hard, good organizational skills, responsibility, determination, and carrying out intentions. At work they will be considered highly ethical. In contrast, their opposite types are reluctant to work hard, sometimes even lazy, disorderly and disorganized, sloppy, and indecisive.

- **E**xtroverts versus Introverts – This dimension distinguishes people who are more likely to be involved in society, talkative, and assertive as opposed to closed, reclusive, shy, and withdrawn types.

- **A**greeable vs. Rude – This dimension differentiates people who are characterized by kindness, a pleasant temperament, a willingness to cooperate, and selflessness versus irritable, rude, cynical, and selfish types.

- **N**on-Neurotic vs. Neurotic – Non-neurotic types are usually emotionally stable and calm, self-confident, and thoughtful in decision-making. In contrast, neurotic types are often irritated, anxious, agitated, and subject to negativity.

These five major personality traits are on a scale or spectrum.[30] They present the limits of the scale. Most of us will be somewhere within the range.

Personality traits can change somewhat over time. However, these are not usually radical changes. An extroverted person will not suddenly become an introvert, although there may be situations where the person is less inclined toward extroversion than at other times.[30]

If we accept that certain traits describe us, we can say that the format of our life's journey will be greatly influenced by them. Let's take someone who is characterized by a neurotic tendency. Neuroticism consists of negative emotion and affects our degree of mental stability. One can assume that neurotically-prone types are more easily affected by stress.

Some studies have shown that not only are these personality types strongly affected by stress, they also *create* stress because, as we have seen, the level of stress is influenced by how we perceive an event. Moreover, these people will have some difficulty managing or coping with the situation.[31]

The good news is that, although a person is prone to neuroticism, they can also be open-minded, extroverted to a degree, and relaxed. These qualities are likely to balance their natural tendency toward stressful situations.

As you see, there is nothing to worry about as there is always a remedy. The correct strategy is to find the way to deal with a stressful situation. To develop your coping skills, first you must identify what it is that creates a feeling of stress within, or in other words, what situations or events cause you to experience stress? When hard at work? When we argue with family members? When we are under economic pressure? Once we compile this inventory, it is important to identify how we dealt with these stressors in the past. Have we repressed them? Did we absorb them? Have we moved on?

We mentioned earlier that there are two ways of coping with stress: problem-based coping and emotion-focused coping.[32] When we choose to deal with stress taking a problem-based approach, our method is pragmatic, and we focus on searching for practical solutions to the problem that is troubling us.

Let us suppose we are dealing with problems in an intimate relationship. Things are strained and we are experiencing increasing symptoms of stress and tension. Utilizing a problem-based approach, we will focus our efforts on finding a couples' or marriage counselor or attend workshops that will help us to better communicate with our spouses.

In an emotion-based approach, we will try to act in ways to lessen the negative emotions we are going through. For example, we go on vacation or, for those of us for whom it is helpful, we go on a shopping spree at a local mall (or an extravagant one in New York!). Each of us will choose the right approach for ourselves.

When we choose to avoid dealing with the situation altogether, we make it worse. Emotional disengagement, a flooding of negative emotions overcome us: ("It's happening again", "I always do the wrong thing", "I can't do anything right." etc.).

Sleeping too much, isolating oneself, or exaggerated distractions (such as the aforementioned shopping spree), not only will not help, but they will also actually make the stressful symptoms worse.

Emotional Resilience

Over the years, I have discovered that there are people born with the right balance of the substances in the brain to effectively deal with stress. These are what we would call "cool" people, who flow with changing reality and take life's vicissitudes in stride. They post Instagram photos showing them surfing, on a ski vacation, taking a bungee jump…in short, they take on every challenge possible. Most of them even enjoy stressful situations. They do not suffer the mental and behavioral anxiety that most of us feel when faced with extreme stress.

The fact is, life is easier for them. Their hormonal and chemical composition is simply more balanced and positive. That's the way they were born. Just as there are people who are born thin and remain so, while others battle with excess weight. In the same manner, there are some people who have an easier time coping with stress. They have an abundance of emotional resilience, an almost inexhaustible supply.

What is the Secret Ingredient of Emotional Resilience?

A study conducted by researchers at Yale University looked at how special military unit soldiers, who went through military survival skills training, are able to cope well with extreme stress.[33]

The idea behind this kind of training is that exposure to extreme stress will enable soldiers to function proficiently on the battlefield. However, what is the mechanism that allows certain soldiers to succeed under extreme battlefield stress? Is it merely a conscious behavioral choice, or is there a biological, brain-related explanation?

These training courses deal with exposure to stress, much like introducing a weakened form of bacterium into the body to improve its immune system (like flu vaccines). The concept is that the body will learn to cope with the condition and strengthen its defenses to successfully fight the virus or bacteria. By the same token, exposure to physical and mental strife and pressure will make soldiers more effective in dangerous and stressful situations.

In the above study the results were intriguing: It turns out that there were high levels of an amino acid called neuropeptide Y (NPY) in every soldier in the special units without exception.

Neuropeptide Y acts as a regulator for memory and enables the anterior regions of the brain to go into action. It is responsible for appetite, learning ability, and blood pressure. Some call it a "natural sedative" or a fire extinguisher for alarm sensors in threat situations because it affects anxiety levels and acts as a buffer against the effects of stress hormones such as norepinephrine (hormones secreted during exposure to stress).

This study is intriguing because it states, almost for the first time, that there is indeed a biochemical structure in the brain (certain levels and compositions of chemicals) that delineate our mental resilience to stressful situations. The question is whether this is an innate ability, or can intensive training improve someone's emotional resilience.

The answer is yes...and yes. First, there are indeed people who are innately capable, and the military is very skilled in identifying them. Second, mental resilience can be enhanced in each of us through integrated physical and mental training.

So why are some of us more naturally resilient than others? The secret has not yet been fully unraveled, although the picture is becoming clearer. Most likely, the "naturals" starting point is higher. Sometimes we may think that when we were children everything was fine and we coped very well with stress, and that the pressures of adult life have made it harder for some of us to cope.

Stock phrases such as, "What doesn't kill you makes you stronger," or "Time heals all wounds," have taken root in society and often have some basis in reality. However, it is undoubtedly true that each of our brains work in a unique manner and each person's life experience affects us in different ways.

In a series of studies conducted by psychologist Jerome Kagan, it was found that in a sampling of sixteen-week-old infants, 20 percent appeared more terrified than the others when exposed to colorful toys placed directly in front of their faces and moved back and forth. These babies can be called *high-reactive* infants.

In comparison, 40 percent of the infants with similar background characteristics remained calm when exposed to the same stimulus and were much less alarmed.[34]

In Kagan's view, the mechanism that created the differences in response was related to the amygdala. In the studies he conducted, it was found that in the frightened infants the circles of fear found in the amygdala showed greater neural activity than the other, calmer infants. These infants have a higher level of fear-related hormones.

It has also been found that the arousal level of those infants susceptible to environmental changes in the brainstem is lower. That is, if they suddenly experience an environment that is somewhat unfamiliar to them, such as, if they wake up and one of their parents is not near them, their immediate response will be shrieking – quite unpleasant to the ear.

It was further found that infants who were frightened and alarmed as infants would probably grow up to be anxious adults (another "good" reason to blame the parents).

To sum up, the answer to why some people are more mentally immune than others lies in our genetic maps, environmental influence, as well as our psychobiological composition. The good news is that, once again, despite everything, there is always hope.

STRATEGIES FOR DEALING WITH STRESS

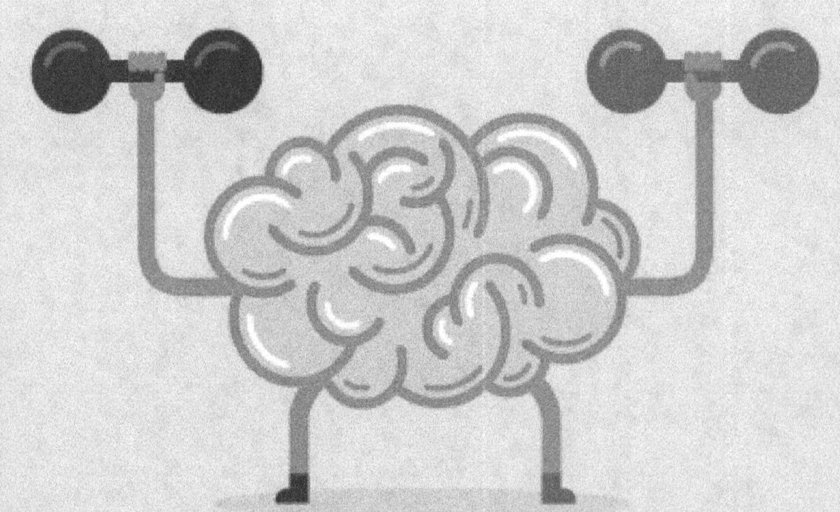

CHAPTER FIVE

STRATEGIES FOR DEALING WITH STRESS

A byword for stress management strategies:
"What doesn't kill me, makes me stronger.",
"If we are doomed to suffer, at least enjoy it."

In this section, I will review the stress management strategies in widespread use today. Some of them will be familiar to you, and some of the tools I present will no doubt be self-evident.

I urge you, dear readers, not to undervalue what you know and to persevere in regular practice. Constant training enables our brain to create new networks of neurons and eventually creates a change in our thinking patterns, replacing defective patterns with new and more effective ones.

Common Treatment Methods

The aim of this sub-chapter is to lay bare to you some common methods of dealing with emotional distress and suffering. Most of the described methods I have experimented with myself.

Naturally, everyone will choose the method that suits

them, but it is important to ascertain that if you decide to be guided by a professional therapist just make sure that the therapist you choose is qualified, with the appropriate license and training. You should also seek recommendations from friends and acquaintances as to the effectiveness of their therapist's treatment.

Remember, not every treatment is suitable for every problem or person, so we often find ourselves trying out a variety of methods until we can find the therapist and treatment method that best suits our needs.

At the core of all these methods is the patient, who is at the center. The role of the therapist is to reflect to the patient the reality as he sees it and to help him improve his level of functioning. The therapist should also provide the patient with tools to deal with what is troubling him or her.

An open interaction between therapist and patient is essential, as is the therapist's capacity to listen and empathize, and the patient's desire to implement the therapist's recommendations.

1. Psychotherapy

Psychotherapy is derived from the world of psychological treatment. "Psycho" in Greek means mind and "therapy" means "treatment." There are many subcategories within Psychotherapy, but it is worth discussing three of these approaches briefly, each of which utilizes different techniques and branches too diverse and detailed to be dealt with in the scope of this book:

The Analytical Approach – This approach focuses on a patient's beliefs, values, and relationships with his or her environment as well as their basic perceptions.

The Psychotherapeutic-Dynamic Approach – This approach attempts to understand the repressed basis of mental distress, that is, the source of distress that occurred in the early years of the patient's life. It is based on the psychoanalytic theory first formulated by Sigmund Freud. This approach is usually effective when it comes to a problem that is generalized and unfocused, such as a vague feeling of emptiness. In such a case, treatment aims at deepening patient understanding and suggesting ways of solving problems through an understanding of complex mental processes.

The Cognitive Behavioral Approach (CBT) – This approach is considered to be the most popular technique in use in recent years. With CBT approach, the focus is on a specific, defined problem and treatment is shorter (studies have shown effective change can take place after as few as ten sessions with a qualified CBT therapist).

CBT treatment focuses on behavioral change in habit and thinking patterns. The method deals with how we think and helps us control and unconditionally accept our thoughts. Many studies show that by accepting our thoughts – whatever they may be – will reduce our feeling of fear.

Several studies have also indicated that the method is effective as an intervention strategy aimed at managing stress in the workplace. The treatment allows employees to acquire cognitive tools that will positively influence their behavioral patterns when in stressful, repetitive situations. CBT, and other therapies such as mindfulness-based meditation, have been found to be very effective in these circumstances.[35]

NLP, (Neuro-linguistic programming) – NLP was developed in the 1970s by Dr. Richard Bandler and Professor John Grinder. The "neuro" value denotes that all behavior is based on neurological processing of the information absorbed by our senses. The "linguistic" value refers to the fact that language is an essential element in organizing our thoughts and communicating with other humans.

"Programming" refers to the assertion that through practice and training you can change how you think, then subsequently act, which affects our neurological system.[36] Note that this method has been criticized by many in the treatment field for failing to comply with scientific requirements for empirical research, such as the need for a control group[36] Despite this criticism, however, the method remains popular and you can find many offers on the Internet for NLP workshops and seminars.

NLP is a stand-alone system and is a training method in and of itself. Practitioners do not necessarily have to be qualified professionals in the field, such as psychologists, doctors, social workers, or other certified psychotherapists. In view of this, although NLP is a feasible option for treatment, it is incumbent on anyone entering NLP treatment to carefully choose his or her counselor or coach and take the limitations of the method into account.

2. Biofeedback

The roots of this method are in the 1960's. The method was first introduced at the founding conference of the Santa Monica Biofeedback Research Association in October 1969. Biofeedback as a therapeutic model and proven technique is based on sensitive electronic instrumentation capable of providing reliable, significant information about the physiological processes. The biofeedback patient gains greater awareness of himself, especially the control and monitoring of his physiological responses. As a result, the patient can learn how to effectively self-regulate.[37]

Imagine that you are connected to sensors in certain areas of your body and that you are sitting in front of a computer screen. When you feel a negative emotion, the device collects the physiological information (such as increased heart rate, brain wave movement, breathing, skin temperature, etc.) and presents it on a graph. After long practice, you can learn how to control these physiological manifestations.

The immediate feedback works on the brain and allows it to learn and inculcate new behaviors and habits. Visual and audio feedback allow the patient to learn for himself how to change his or her reactions when in different stress situations. This method is based on empirical studies and has been shown to be effective in regulating stress. Equally important, it can be applied in clinics with qualified therapists as well as in the workplace.

Some therapists, after professional analysis, choose to utilize two treatment methods together, such as CBT and biofeedback. This method aids rational people who seek "logical" explanations for the tension they are suffering that is causing them chronic pain. The explanation for this includes visual and audio representations which help the patient understand that there is a reason for their problem, and more importantly, that there is a solution.

An assortment of other treatment methods exists: (art therapy, drama, movement, the plastic arts, music therapy, and more). These are designed to induce relaxation in stressful situations.

3. Mindfulness

It is seven in the morning. I woke up about a quarter of an hour ago and my body needs to start my daily practice. My mind prompts me to take a deep breath and enter a state of quiet consciousness.

Some people believe (and I am one of them) that mindfulness is a world-shaking concept that enables everyone to take a "time out" from their stressful lives and bring equilibrium and serenity into them. The ability to develop mindfulness, or in other words to become attuned to what is going on inside us at this very moment, clarifies and categorizes what I truly love and need in my life, and what things are less important for me.

The definition of mindfulness is attentive awareness or unconditional listening to our inner selves. The guiding principle is spiritual observation of what is happening only at this very moment and no other. The emphasis is on the present moment, unconditionally, and most importantly, without judgment. It sounds complex, but the fact is, it is not.

Think of how many times during the day you go through an experience at a particular moment and immediately judge it as good or bad? It turns out that it's almost always...

As human beings, we were born judgmental. Perhaps judgment comes from our need to protect ourselves and what we believe, but judgment is also a source of many problems in human relationships. How many times have you gone shopping at the supermarket and complained to yourself – or to other people in the queue that the cashier was terribly slow? It probably has happened quite a bit.

We often make judgments in situations where we generally do not have enough reliable and valid information about what is actually going on. Our lack of good information is complicated by our personally held beliefs, which in many cases may be wrong and far from the truth. The cashier you complained about may be preoccupied with thinking how she is going to be able to buy things for the coming holiday when she does not currently have the money. Or, she may be worried about her son getting in trouble at school, and so on.

With mindfulness, we train the mind to look around us at every moment, both emotionally and physically, without the need to change anything. Once we look at a given moment and just be in it completely, and don't have the urge to change it, our pre-judgment of the situation will vanish.

Jon Kabat-Zinn is an American professor emeritus of medicine and the creator of the Stress Reduction Clinic and the Center for Mindfulness in Medicine, Health Care, and Society at the University of Massachusetts Medical School. When he was a student at MIT, he presented his mindfulness program in a series of eight sessions. Each session is about two hours and encompassed mindfulness, meditation, and thought training.

The practice is designed so that we first become fully cognizant of the sensations in our bodies at any given moment – the thoughts, feelings, and actions. This step helps us through unconditional and nonjudgmental awareness to replace old habits with new ones.

The success of the program requires daily practice that starts out at five minutes a day and builds to forty-five minutes for the most advanced among us. Based on the principles outlined by Kabat-Zinn, MBSR (Mindfulness-based Stress Reduction) was developed to address stress and anxiety[38-40].

When I first read about MBSR, I didn't grasp its true significance. However, after constant practice which began as natural curiosity, I eventually came to the conclusion that today's world is all about grabbing and capturing our attention.

The frenetic pace of happenings, the constantly evolving technology, and our need to be always and instantaneously "in the know" – take us out of the present moment and does not even allow us to fully experience and appreciate the great tasting sandwich that we wolfed down a second ago.

Speaking of the sandwich, I have noticed that I usually prefer to eat while doing something else, such as watching TV or reading the news in a paper or on my cellphone. My attention is not focused on experiencing the taste of the sandwich. Sometimes I don't even recall what I ate because I was so busy with other things.

Have you ever driven home and suddenly found yourself in your driveway because you let your mind start to ruminate? If you were to calculate the time you spent with your thoughts wandering to distant shores, I am certain you would find that more than half the time you spent thinking about things that had nothing to do with what you were doing at the moment.

One of the insights that changed my life came from a class I attended on the topic of mindfulness. The lecturer, a man who had devoted his life to the subject, told us about the incurable illness his wife was dealing with. She, and everyone else around her, knew that she would never recover. In a joint decision he and his wife decided to study mindfulness.

They delved into the subject and understood that mental suffering occurs mainly because we so very much want to change a certain reality. When there is conflict between what we want and what exists, we suffer as a result. Our suffering is further exacerbated when we also desire to escape from the existing reality and somehow change it.

Understanding that this is the central source of suffering can change our perception. If we understand the reason, we will see that we are not a victim of reality. Things happen and you can't change the fact that they happened. We need to understand that we are not victims, and that these life lessons have their own trajectory. If we truly understand this, we will no longer try to change reality because it is a given and is immutable. From this point on, it is important we understand what led us here, and how we can live without judgment, and consequently with less suffering and frustration.

When I tried to explain to a friend how to practice mindfulness, his initial response was, "It sounds too simplistic and spiritual to me."

I insisted he should try. After a few days, he told me of the difficulties he had while trying to practice. The frequent response from beginners is that they can't concentrate, and their thoughts are knocking constantly on the door of their mind.

It is a common response and from my experience you should let it go, just do it, don't fight your stream of thoughts. In a few sessions you will learn to enjoy it, and from my experience it will be faster than you think. Meditation requires readiness, acceptance of self, and the acceptance of feelings of suffering and frustration we experience.

The challenge is self-discipline, perseverance, and knowing that it will take time to reach a state of understanding, insight, and awareness. If you persist, after a few months you will see positive results. It is not easy to ignore everything around us – spouse, children, work, television, smartphone, etc. It is easier to pay attention to these stimuli rather than stand aside and concentrate on our inner selves.

Practicing mindfulness is a very effective way of life, especially in reducing stress. When we are stressed, our attention is focused mainly on repetitive thinking, rumination, self-criticism, and judgment, none of which contributes to our sense of well-being.

Through practice of mindfulness we learn to focus our awareness on what is happening now, at this moment. Our breath and body are the anchors that are with us always, and hone in on the moment. We are used to trying to control everything in our lives. We are captive to the basic misconception that control must inevitably lead to a desired outcome for us.

This attempt to control everything in our environment results in suffering and frustration. There will always be a gap between what we hoped would occur and what really happens. Such disappointment can lead us to question our worth, our abilities, and even our relationships with those around us. The doubt and insecurity associated with these feelings only further aggravates our suffering.

How to Practice Mindfulness – Step by Step

1. First, focus your attention on what is happening to you, whether an action, a thought, or a feeling.

2. In the second stage, focus only on this moment. Even if thoughts run through your mind and you are thinking about what happened last night and what will happen later. Gently try to focus on what is happening RIGHT now. You will be aware of many thoughts. Allow the thoughts running through your mind to pass by without judgment, and without any effort.

3. Now focus on the given moment without judgment. If judgment comes, let it pass without delving into it or attaching any meaning to it.

Studies have shown that mindfulness contributes to reducing stress levels. In a meta-analytic study in the field, it was found that those subjects practicing mindfulness (the treatment group) significantly reduced stress symptoms compared with subjects in the control group.[42]

What, then, is the mechanism affected by practicing mindfulness, and how does it work? Findings show that long-term practice is associated with changes in neuroplasticity in certain areas of the brain, for example in the anterior cingulate cortex. This area is part of the limbic system in the brain. It receives stimuli from the environment and helps with emotional and cognitive processing.

When practicing mindfulness meditation, the anterior cingulate cortex becomes much more active. It enables us to focus attention on the given moment despite conflicting information flowing to us during mindfulness practice such as thoughts, external stimuli and feelings. This allows us to regulate and diminish the background noise.[43]

Another study of sixteen mindfulness practitioners found that after eight weeks of exercise, the concentration of the gray matter in the left hippocampal in the brain increased.[44] (The gray matter is made up of a scattered network of areas in the brain that are believed to be involved in information processing. It is rich in nerve cell bodies and is gray in color. The increase in gray matter in a particular area indicates a functional improvement in that area. In the same study it was noted that gray matter concentration had also increased in other brain areas related to memory, learning, emotion regulation, and other processes.)

In conclusion, it is possible to say these studies definitively point to the effectiveness of mindfulness treatment (MBSR). The method succeeds in reducing the level of anxiety, as well as diminish extraneous thoughts and rumination. In addition, practicing mindfulness gives one a feeling of acceptance and self-compassion.[45]

Strategies for Stress Management

Appreciate What you Have – Take Nothing for Granted

Expression of this age-old strategy can be found in almost every book that deals with positive thinking. It seems obvious, but it is difficult to apply in reality. It is important to set aside a time when we can sit and process what we appreciate in our lives and think about what we have that is not self-evident.

Have you ever thought about how you breathe, see, or feel? These senses are not self-evident. Gratitude for what exists and not for what doesn't, allows us to make genuine change. The question arises as to why this strategy must be learned, and why it is not inborn in us? In my opinion, this is the result of Western secular education. Religious and people of faith will most probably adopt this strategy more easily than others, as these are principles inherent in faith and the commandments.

A study conducted at the University of California found that people who worked on a daily basis to cultivate gratitude and appreciation experienced a marked improvement in their mood, energy, and physical state.[46] Physically, this manifests itself by way of a substantial reduction in the amount of cortisol secretion in the brainstem.

Another method for dealing with stress that has been found to be effective in many cases, is to imagine the opposite situation. Picture how your life would be without what you have achieved so far? Even if the physical and spiritual capital you have amassed so far does not seem significant to you, you have done it with your own hands and worthy of preservation.

Also, can you imagine your life without the presence of some of the people around you? Without a roof over your head, without friends, or a job? Even if sometimes these things annoy us, they are part of our lives and situations arise where they are very meaningful to us. If that is so, it is worth pausing for a moment, at least once a day, to thank ourselves and the world we live in. To be thankful for the good and the less good in our lives.

Avoid asking, "What if?", "What if I don't pass the test?", "What if the meeting is a failure?", "What if I fail to give an effective lecture or presentation?" Our brain is just waiting for all these thought patterns and fears. It is fuel for the fire and the road to stress in a field of flaming thorns is very short indeed. But take heart. Who said this black-and-white scenario would actually play out?

One thing is clear: when we spend so much time wondering what will happen, we spend much less time on taking actions that may calm us down and keep our stress level in check.

In this context, it is important for me to mention the familiar *Sliding Doors* theory from a 1998 film of the same name directed by Peter Howitt (the film was inspired by Krzysztof Kieslowski's 1987 film *Blind Chance*).

A brief plot description: Helen (played by actress Gwyneth Paltrow), who is fired from her job at a public relations firm in London, rushes to catch a subway train in the London Underground. From here, the plot diverges into two parallel worlds. The film raises the question, "What if, at some point,

I was to choose differently?" The answer is clear – we can never know what would have happened.

A similar, well-known theory is the "butterfly effect." According to this theory, a butterfly's fluttering wings make minuscule changes in the atmosphere that cause increasingly greater changes in the atmosphere, leading even to the force of a hurricane.

That is to say, if we were to make choices, even slightly different from what we actually choose to do, there would be momentous and unexpected changes in our lives.

In conclusion, we can say that drifting into reflection on our choices does not help calm us, it only increases our stress. None of us have the ability to know what would have happened if we had chosen one way and not another. It is better to live in the present and deal with what exists.

Adopt Positive Thinking

Positive thoughts help reduce stress. On the other hand, research shows that negative thoughts can actually shorten our live span.

What happens when we are flooded with negativity?

Negative thoughts damage our body cells by causing them to age faster. The source of this phenomenon lies in molecules called telomeres.

A study by a group of researchers at the University of California found that telomere length is affected by, among other things, chronic stress. The study was carried out with a group of two hundred thirty-nine healthy women over a period of one year.

By studying the length of the telomeres in the women's bodies, it was found that after exposure to stress factors, the length of the telomeres changed and they were significantly shorter.[47]

How does this mechanism work and how is it related to chronic stress?

The telomere is the tip on chromosomes that contain hereditary material inside the nucleus of the cell. Just as the aglet, the plastic tip of a shoe lace protects it, so does the telomere protect the chromosome. Each chromosome has two ends and, therefore, two telomeres.

When the body is in a state of stress it secretes powerful stress hormones within a short period of time. The brain perceives this as a danger signal and raises the level of readiness in the cells. The body is thus prepared for "war," with all available resources mobilized.

The level of telomerase, which is the enzyme responsible for the elongating the telomere, also increases. When stress lasts for a long period, the body responds accordingly: Telomeres are damaged and shortened, and hence, the path to various diseases is diminished and aging is accelerated.

Studies have looked at the physical reactions of people categorized as pessimistic and found that their telomere length is indeed shorter.[48, 49] It turns out, however, that not only pessimistic people produce negative thoughts, it happens to all of us. Although we try to limit our thoughts on other problems and concerns around us, it causes us to focus on them.

Try this little experiment on yourself for a moment. Try not to think of a pink rabbit in the next few minutes, try hard not to think about it. Take a minute and write down how many times you thought of a pink rabbit, even though you tried not to. I'm certain you pictured a pink rabbit many, many times.

This phenomenon is called "ironic errors of thought,"[50] i.e., situations where the more we try to suppress a certain thought, the more our brain will focus on it, no matter how hard we try not to do so.

An ironic error is exacerbated when our mental control is weak, which happens in ongoing stressful situations, such as chronic illness, physical pain, gloom, depression, anxiety, etc.

Edgar Allan Poe wrote a short essay about self-destructiveness entitled, *The Imp of the Perverse*, which makes us do things precisely because we tried so hard to avoid doing them.[51, 52] The imp is often found in our lives. As much as we try to shake it off, we are going to lose the battle.

What can we do about this?

By consciously choosing positive thoughts, we can refocus our attention. When everything is going well, and your mood is good, it's easy. But when nothing goes well, when your mood is poor, and your mind is flooded with negative thoughts, it is a daunting challenge.

When you are feeling negative emotions, try to scan

the events that happened that day and identify a moment or a few positive moments that occurred. Even if you don't think anything positive happened, you will come up with something. First, the very fact that you woke up and you are healthy, is a joyous, positive thing.

Find something positive in your day and concentrate on it. It doesn't matter how small and insignificant it may seem to you at that moment. Focus on it, write it down, and try to visualize it. Try to share this moment with those close to you. When you follow these steps, you will sense that this moment was meaningful.

When we are in a stressful situation, most of us carry out a repetitive pattern of action. Usually this pattern consists of two assumptions: the first is that something will happen, and the second is that what happens will be bad. One way to deal with these feelings is to take a pen and paper or open a Word document on your computer and write at least three reasons why what we fear may not happen at all.

This very action may immediately reduce the feeling of stress. Your thinking shifted from, "I'm sure it will happen," to "maybe it will, but maybe not." Now think for a moment what will happen if the result is less than good, what good things might come of it anyway.

Now your thinking will no longer just be, "something is coming, and it will be bad," but "maybe it will or may not happen, and even if it isn't good, chances are something good may come out of it."

If we adopt this strategy, we can change thinking patterns that have become automatic. From a situation where we are accustomed to thinking that we have control over the results and they are destined to be bad, we will come to understand that the world is complex, reality is dynamic and flowing, and our control over events is minimal, if we have any at all. Even if things do happen as we fear they might, our ability to deal with them will be better.

Don't work 24/7!

Long working hours, endless tasks, and emails pouring into your mailbox means constant exposure to stressors. Not only do these things generate stress, but they also change the way our brain works.

No one wants to feel that he or she is replaceable, so many of us (often without our being aware of it) become workaholics. In a competitive economy where everyone is vying for good jobs, people feel the need to prove themselves nonstop, so that they can feel needed and that their workplace is secure.

This mindset has become so extreme that many employees feel the need to be up-to-the-minute on work issues, answering phones and emails, even while on vacation.

Our self-image, identity, and worth are most often defined by our work. We are used to thinking that everything we have achieved, such as getting our children into the "right" activities or going on our vacation in Tuscany, has been made possible by our work, so we have to do whatever it takes to preserve it.

I'm not saying that it's not true. Work is extremely important, but we have somewhat forgotten in recent years that to be good workers, we also need leisure time with ourselves and our families.

In the past it was enough that we ended the work day and left the office, but today's technological advancements do not allow us to completely break away. We don't have to be physically in the workplace at all. The computer and the cellphone make us available virtually all the time, night or day. At almost every social gathering I attend, I hear people complaining about working too hard.

So what can you do? Disconnect!

You have to decide and take action by going offline for distinct periods of time. Believe me, nothing untoward will happen. You will not lose your job if you don't answer someone at that very moment. Not just on weekends, but *definitely* on weekends.

If you are sitting down at dinner with the family, turn off your phone or at least put it on silent mode. I adopted a method and gave my partners and employees my wife's mobile number and my home phone number. If something terrible happens, god forbid, I know they can always find me, even if I'm not personally available.

Even during the work day, give yourself a few moments or even half-hour periods when you are not busy reading emails, answering text messages, or talking on the phone. You'll be surprised how refreshing it can be. Share your decisions with the people closest to you, including your employees. Ask them not to disturb you on weekends, except under extraordinary circumstances. Once in place, you can gradually extend these time-out periods.

It is important that you set a personal example and avoid

interrupting others during their after work hours except in an emergency. This reciprocity will be greatly appreciated and will help you to build a positive and supportive system with your colleagues or employees and their families.

Cut down your exposure time on social networks

According to data gathered by Apple, the average person uses their smartphone about eighty times a day or about twenty-nine thousand times in a year. This figure illustrates how smartphones have become such an integral part of our lives, or in essence, the real manager of our lives.

Apple smartphone users will be able to check this out for themselves in their new release version. Apple has added a feature that lets every user receive data analyzing use of their smartphone.

In your next casual conversation with those close to you, ask them what the importance is of a smartphone in their lives. You will be surprised to hear (or perhaps not) that many of them tell you how vital their phone is to them and that they cannot conceive of their lives without it. But here's the rub: along with the admittedly miraculous benefits the smartphone offers us, it also can produce anxiety that leads to serious stress.

I'm sure every one of you have, at least once if not more, forgotten your smartphone and couldn't remember where you left it.

Studies show that in these moments, blood pressure rises, the pulse accelerates, and the brain interprets the condition as a threat, with all its alarming implications.

Our need to be available around the clock leads to chronic stress. The sympathetic nervous system, which responds to external stressors, works around the clock and so do other systems in the body. The body is in a state of constant alert to dangers, like a man lost in the Amazon Rainforest.

The smartphone is indisputably one of the greatest distractors of attention in our lives. It is not only the device itself, of course, but also in large part the myriad of applications installed on it. How many of you use at least one of the social networking apps such as Facebook, WhatsApp, or Instagram?

Try a little experiment. Send a WhatsApp to a friend. How do you feel when the double blue check marks next to your message have not appeared after a minute or two?

These feelings have a name and are classified as new psychological disorders. For example: Nomophobia is defined as the fear of being without your smartphone or having access to it, and the Phantom ringing syndrome (when you think your phone is ringing but it is not) is the fear of not being updated. These phenomena increase the sense of pressure and suffocation we experience in Western society and modern life.

You can try all kinds of ways to help you get rid of your smartphone. For example, buy a phone black or white in color – they are considered less tempting. Or have one that will remind you to disconnect from social networks. It is important to remember that the best way is to find the right balance.

During your leisure moments, try to disconnect from your phones at least from eight in the evening (off or on silent mode). Be assured that someone can find you in an emergency, and even if you are not updated to the last second during the night, nothing terrible will happen. It is preferable that applications like Facebook should not be on a smartphone in the first place, but only on a computer.

Remember that although many people say that the smartphone reassures them, the opposite is probably true. We are flooded with information and stimuli. Often the rate of information flow exceeds the brain's ability to absorb and process it emotionally.

That's why relentless use of a smartphone can lead to "psycho-digital" disorders, causing stress, and impairing our quality of life.

Aim for a balanced lifestyle: good nutrition, adequate sleep, and exercise

Here are Some Recommendations:

Cut down on caffeine

Caffeine promotes the production of adrenaline that, during periods of stress, is a source of "fight or flight," the reaction mechanism that makes us either freeze or fight. It is advisable to moderate caffeine intake found in cola, red bull, and coffee or tea. The daily recommendation is to consume at most four hundred mg of caffeine, equivalent to about four cups of coffee per day.

Sleeping habits

Quality sleep is important for refreshing the brain. Do not fall asleep with the television blaring in the background, and do not have a phone nearby. Sleep quality can be improved first and foremost by having comfortable sleeping conditions, a proper pillow, blanket, appropriate low lighting, and quiet all surrounding you.

Good quality sleep is essential to normal daily functioning. It is also recommended to practice meditation about half an hour before bed, using one of your preferred methods. Try to establish a regular ritual – your private sleeping ritual. To get ready for sleep, do the following:

1. Place your tongue on the upper palate, just behind the front teeth. – Try to leave it there throughout the entire routine.

2. Breathe out from your mouth – one very long exhale.

3. Keep your mouth closed and inhale through your nose for four or five seconds to take more oxygen into the body.

4. Hold your breath for seven seconds to allow oxygen to penetrate the bloodstream.

5. Open your mouth and exhale for eight or ten seconds to slow your heart rate and release more carbon dioxide from your lungs.

6. Repeat this several times and most likely you will awaken refreshed in the morning.

In short: inhale through your nose for four seconds, hold your breath for seven seconds, and exhale through your nose for eight seconds.

Proper Nutrition

Neurogenesis. The aim is to create new neurons in the brain. For years, it was thought that no new nerve cells formed as we age, but it is now known that neurogenesis also takes place on a limited basis throughout our adult life as well.

To date, evidence has only been found in two areas of the mammalian brain: in the hippocampus and the olfactory bulb.

To date, there is no evidence of neurogenesis taking place in the human cortex. The hippocampus is located in the lower part of the brain, adjacent to the spinal cord. It is responsible for a variety of important functions such as memory, orientation in space, mood, emotions, and more.

The formation of neurons in the brain occurs mainly during fetal development. At this time, billions of stem cells are created, compared to an adult brain that produces perhaps seven hundred new cells a day. The fact is, by age fifty, all the hippocampal nerve cells we were born with will have been replaced by new nerve cells.

A researcher by the name of Tracey Shors has found that not only does neuron production continue in later life, but we can also control the rate of production and the length of time that neurons will function in the brain.[48]

Zainuddin and Dr. S. Thuret, among others, investigated the relationship between nutrition, mental health, and neurogenesis[53] Based on research in the field, it is clear that new hippocampal nerve cells can be affected by nutrition.

It was further found that depressed individuals had a lower rate of the creation of new cells. When depressed persons were treated with antidepressants, new nerve cell production rates increased and the symptoms of depression were reduced.

In humans, sleep deprivation, stress, and aging reduce the production of new nerve cells, while learning, sex, and running, speed up the process.

Another important issue is dietary habits. Nutrition affects the level of neurogenesis, which in turn affects our memory and our emotional state. It appears that reducing calorie intake by about 25 percent, having a long break between meals, and consuming food that requires chewing, will promote the production of new nerve cells and contribute to improving our mental state, even in cases of depression.

Also, consumption of flavonoids (pigments found in foods like blueberries, dark chocolate, citrus, legumes, soybeans, and tea), Omega-3 (abundant in salmon, avocado, and walnuts), and moderate consumption of red wine is very helpful. In contrast, saturated, high-fat foods will impair cell growth and cause worsening of depressive symptoms.

Exercise

Studies in recent years indicate the great importance of physical activity, not only in maintaining your health (improving cardiovascular endurance, and strengthening the neural system, the skeleton, and muscles), but also the important effect of physical activity on the brain and its function at any age.

Researchers in the field maintain that strenuous exercise helps the cognitive development of our brains, just as the need to flee contributed to the development of our ancestors' brains and aided in their survival.

How does physical activity affect cognitive development? Exercise is essential for brain development and it affects its development by way of a number of mechanisms including: Increased oxygen consumption, increased secretion of neurotransmitters, and increased secretion of neurotrophins.

During exercise, oxygen consumption and blood flow increase.[54] This allows oxygen and blood to flow into the muscles, including the brain. In this way it was discovered that new blood vessels are created in a process called angiogenesis in the brain.

And so, the oxygen uptake improves in the blood in areas of the brain that are essential for cognitive tasks.

A second mechanism enables physical activity to increase levels of neurotransmitters, such as serotonin and norepinephrine.

This increase facilitates the processing of information in the brain. A large amount of these materials allow for more efficient "wiring" of the neuronal network in the brain, making communication and transmission of the chemical messages between the various nerve cells and the different regions of the brain more efficient.

Over time, physical exercise results in brain training, which means that the number of brain connections will increase and so will its function.[55]

The third mechanism causes an increase in secretion of

neurotrophins during physical exercise. Neurotrophins are the proteins responsible for brain tissue and are extremely important in producing the substances that nerve cells need during our childhood development.

The role of neurotrophins is also to preserve brain cells, and to ensure their survival at an older age when the rate of brain cell production is decreasing. It has been shown that although the rate of production decreases as we age, there are still areas of the brain where new nerve cells are growing.

The mechanism responsible for this works, among other things, by way of the neurotrophins. It follows that a higher secretion of these substances will not only help maintain existing brain cells, but they will also stimulate the creation of new cells in later age.[56]

The brain of ancient humankind required physical activity not only to avert danger, but also to evolve as human beings. The human brain today also requires physical activity. Although people today rarely have to physically escape from danger, they do need skills such as decision-making at an effective pace, and information storage to continually cope with the many stimuli in their environment.

It has been borne out that people who are physically active all their lives also have good cognitive skills. Some of us feel we have a real need for physical activity, that it is a requirement of our brain.

But what about those who don't feel the need? The answer probably lies in our genetics. Research on this subject is ongoing daily and the relevant genes have yet to have been fully mapped, but in my estimation we will soon be able to understand the genetic mapping that makes some of us want physical activity and others who are really not interested in it.

Genetic studies can help the "couch potatoes among us." In my experience, you just have to get started, slowly at first, and in a controlled manner. In this way, the mechanisms we described earlier will come into play and over time, our brains will develop a need for a greater amount of these substances.

The cycle will begin to feed upon itself and will keep us going with exercise. I learned first-hand, and I frequently give up an hour of sleep in order to engage in physical activity. There are many others who do the same.

Posture and Breathing

Research shows that there is a connection between our posture and our mental state. Sound strange? Not really. An upright posture affects our emotional state and can reduce feelings of sadness, as well as lower anxiety and stress levels.

Imagine for a moment that you wish to improve your cardiorespiratory endurance. How do you do that? The answer is simple. You run at the gym on the track, on the beach, or along the side of a road.

Your brain needs exercising and one of the important elements of exercise is posture. A particular posture will be related to a particular emotion. For example, if we sit in a comfortable armchair in a relaxing place and breathe deeply and slowly, this action will be linked in the brain to a state of calm.

This is exciting news. So far, studies have shown that muscle relaxation helps reduce stress,[57] and that dancing can make you feel happy. The effect of posture on our emotions is a new topic for study.

Interesting research done in 2010 by Colombia University and Harvard[58] found that two minutes of low-power sitting, raised cortisol levels (the hormone secreted during stress and anxiety). In addition it was found that low-power sitting is linked with a sense of powerlessness. On the other hand in high power sitting, lower cortisol levels were found. The mood of subjects in high - power posture was more positive, and they felt better about themselves.

In a study led by Dr. Tal Shafir and her associates in 2013,[59] it was found that mobility and posture, and even the mere image of erect posture, will enhance our emotional state, and link it to that specific posture.

Shafir understood that body posture can be a tool for regulating our emotions, and even a tool for diagnosing the emotional state of those around us.

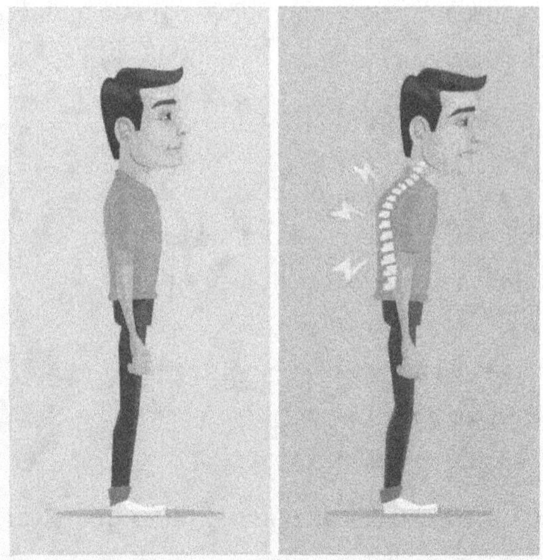

Regulate Your Breathing:

Breathing is undoubtedly the most important activity in our lives and paradoxically it is also probably the simplest, instinctive, and most automated. That's just the way it is for human beings. Anything that is self-evident in our lives does not take up much room in our conscious mind. However, breathing is actually the most important and fundamental element in stress reduction.

Let me explain the significance of breathing to our physical and mental health. As we breathe, the act of itself conveys to the brain a calming effect called a "relaxation response." The brain, in turn, transmits a signal to the central nervous system to relax.

The body responds accordingly: the heart rate slows

down, blood pressure stabilizes, the muscles relax, and breathing becomes slower and slower. If we practice relaxed breathing for twenty to thirty seconds, we will accustom the body to a more tranquil state, thus freeing our brain from the "fight or flight" response that can be evoked by stress.

There are many types of breathing exercises. I have chosen to present to you an abdominal breathing exercise that in my mind is simple, but definitely effective:

Step 1 – Prepare yourself by sitting upright in a chair, in a comfortable yoga position or reclining. Take two deep breaths and close your eyes.

Step 2 – Focus your attention on breathing. Observe how cooler air enters when you breathe in and gets warmer when you breathe out. Do this several times. This will allow you to focus on the present moment, despite the tendency to dwell on reflective thoughts.

Step 3 – Breathing technique: Take ten breaths as follows: Breathe in deeply through your nose. Place one hand in the center of your abdomen. Feel it fill with air as you breathe in. Breathe in deeply until you feel like you cannot take in more air. Pause for a moment before releasing the air very slowly. The exhale should take twice as long as the inhalation rate. To begin, I recommend breathing into a count of four, pause for a second and then slowly exhale to a count of eight. Do this ten to twelve times.

Perform this exercise at least three or four times daily. Afterwards, note how you feel.

Thinking Change

Tina Seelig[60] in her book, *Ingenius*, argues that how we respond to problems depends, among other things, on our internal characteristics and the external forces that act upon us.

Internal characteristics include our knowledge, imagination, and most importantly our approach to life. The external characteristics or forces are our immediate and more distant environment: family, work, friends and colleagues, nature, culture, resources, and even how failure is perceived in our society.

In Japanese culture, for example, failure is a humiliating disaster. In other cultures, failure leads to an examination of our actions with the main goal of fixing what went wrong so it may not happen the next time.

How does this relate to our issues? We can alter our way of automatic thinking by deciding to change our perspective on the problems and challenges we face. Once we do that, we redefine the way we look at the problem. Practice and drill will definitely influence a change in our way of thinking.

When we are faced with a disturbing problem, an important principle is to formulate the right question. We must make certain not to limit the range of freedom in the drafting of the question.

An example I came upon in the *Harvard Business Review* (HBR)[61] was an article in the January 2017 issue. Suppose you own a residential building and the tenants keep complaining that the elevator is old and excruciatingly slow.

Most of us would focus on the technical problem itself. That is, they will recommend replacing the elevator with a new one, upgrading the system, or changing the motor, etc. These solutions are based on the defined problem: the elevator is too slow.

When the complaint was addressed to someone whose way of thinking was different, his proposal for a solution was different: the installation of a mirror in the elevator. The idea is that time is relative and if people are given something to engage their attention, they will spend a moment or two or even more gazing into the mirror, so that the length of time spent in the elevator will no longer be relevant.

This example is interesting because the solution does not improve the speed of the elevator, but in fact, the number of complaints were significantly reduced. The hypothesis is that the focus should be on the experience itself (it is not for nothing that our attention is drawn to looking into mirrors and watching TV screens).

Even if we are stuck, discouraged, stressed out, or troubled by a problem, it is important to remember that there is more than one way to solve it.

The range of solutions is flexible and broad and includes many options that we are not always aware of. The problem is that we tend to characterize and analyze the reality around us based on an acquired set of concepts and are much influenced by past experience. This greatly limits our way of thinking.

Everything depends on your perspective. We choose what to focus on, what to ignore, what is important and what is not, and this way of thinking tends to narrow our choices, limiting us to making a comfortable, familiar solution that is not always the optimal one.

A simple practice will enable us to view reality through a wider lens. We can use the people around us to practice asking the right questions, and not necessarily the ones we are used to asking.

Which tools will aid us in adopting new ways of thinking?

Normalizing Emotion

In Buddhist thought it is customary to state that if there is a problem and it has a solution then why worry? And conversely, if there is a problem and it has no solution…then why worry? The message here is that worry has no operative role and is, in fact, a sensory warning of potentially dangerous situations. We tend not to properly process these sensors of concern. To return the sensors to normal, you can use several tools:

- **Perspective** – Think of yourself as part of something bigger. Every person is a private entity, but also part of a group, state, and society. Everyone is coping, not just me. The difference between human beings is not the power and the scale of the problems, but their individual level of resilience to deal with them. At the end of the day all of us have worries. Taking things in proportion and in context will make the difference.

- **Proportion** – "It's not that bad." Try to look at the situation a little from the side and try to think what you can learn from it. It can be an opportunity for change and perhaps for improvement. In most cases, it is not an existential crisis, but only one that is perceived as existential…and there is a profound difference.

> **Alternatives** – Look for ways to change the existing situation. There are always varied options and, in most cases, change can be achieved.

> **Faith** – It is important to believe that there is a solution and that any crisis that creates worry can be resolved. Sometimes the solution requires multiple and varied resources, but they are certainly attainable.

> **Going through the emotions** – It is helpful to summarize the day by compiling a list of your concerns. Why were you worried?
> What caused the worry and how powerfully did you experience the feeling of worry? Is it a repetitive feeling or a new one? Was there really a need to worry? Often, we will find that we were worrying for nothing.

> **Ventilation of Emotions** – It is useful and desirable to share your concerns with colleagues, friends, and family. Merely sharing and describing your concern aloud – including the explanation of reasons for the concern – will immediately reduce its impact and intensity. Concerns usually do not have an objective measurement, but rather a subjective one.
> The intensity of concerns depends largely on their

processing. Ventilating emotions by talking about them will help you to see things in the proper perspective.

- **A Balanced Lifestyle and Daily Routine** – Even when worries are a large part of your life, you must set and maintain a daily routine. Routine will make worrying a smaller portion of your day. Appropriate nutrition and exercise are extremely important. Exercise, intensive and otherwise, allows you to concentrate on the physical movements and causes a release of consciousness, even if temporary, from obsessive thoughts and worries.

- **Manage the crisis, do not let the crisis manage you** – even if it is an objective crisis that indeed deserves concern, the situation can be addressed. It would be accurate to define crisis as an opportunity to change and improve how we behave or think.

  Instead of dwelling on the crisis, its consequences and worry about possible worst results, it would be better to think of a solution and alternatives. Focusing your thought and energy on the process and implementation of a solution will be helpful.

  Identifying the sources of the crisis and recruiting a team of advisers to help prepare a crisis management plan will enable you to understand that it can be managed and even "gotten out of."

  There is always a solution. Sometimes different resources such as time and money will be needed, but there is always a solution.

> **Professional Tools** – Professional advice is desirable, if needed. Counseling can be specific to content area, but it can be on the cognitive level as well. Sometimes we are encased in a haze of thoughts that make it hard for us to see the light by ourselves. Professional counseling (mentoring, psychotherapy, etc.) can certainly help.

Exercises to Help you Relax

Professor Ian Robertson in his book: *The Stress Test: How Pressure Can Make You Stronger and Sharper* (12) and the blog he posts[62] offers a simple exercise that helps reduce tension when facing a stressful situation, such as an important presentation or critical meeting:

Hold a small squeezable ball in your right palm. Crush the ball in your hand for forty-five seconds with a fifteen second rest interval. Do this several times. This triggers the left lobe of the brain that is responsible for a sense of challenge and a good mood. You will feel better in the moment.

Other exercises that I have found to be very effective:

- Sit in an upright position (see recommendations in Sub-chapter 7 Posture and Breathing). Erect posture conveys to the brain confidence in a situation.
- Treat the situation with excitement (positive) rather than stress (negative). When stress is classified as excitement, there is a reduction in pulse levels, which can indicate a reduction in stress level.

In work situations where you need to manage an important project, write up a new work plan. It is highly recommended to break down each complex task into a list of simple actions. In my personal experience, a complex task seems much simpler when deconstructed in this way. This method allows our brain to categorize the execution of the sub-tasks as success. This sense of success releases the dopamine hormone, which has an effect of reducing stress and diminishing a bad mood.

Recently, as I was driving to a meeting, I listened to song on the radio. It was by a favorite band of mine, Imagine Dragons with their hit *Believer*. What got my attention was that not only was the band doing the song, but also a huge group of thousands of people participating in a mass-singing social event called "Koolulam". If you click on the appropriate link on YouTube you will see this amazing phenomenon.

"Koolulam" is a social musical venture in which hundreds, and sometimes thousands, of people of different colors, genders, and ages come together to sing one song at the same time (the variation is slightly different from the original song, but it is also unique).

When I first heard it sung this way, I had an emotional feeling that is hard to describe in words. A combination of peacefulness, joy, and serenity filled my spirit for the first time in a long while. The effect of this song on me was no less than the effect of a chemical pill that I would take to improve my mood.

Listening to music

How does it happen that music affects us and our brains?

Music has an impact on humans because it is an alternative to language. Music has fixed patterns and that is why when we listen to rhythmic music our tendency is to move in concert with it.

Imagine that from now on at every session or meeting you will play music. Think about it and try it. I promise you, you will be surprised by the results.

Music also operates on our emotions and connects to our feelings. Music links up with areas of our brain, which then translates into sensations. The scale of feeling is wide, ranging from great excitement to crying.

It is well-known that pregnant women often play music for the fetus within their womb. The music gives the woman sensations that secrete hormones that reach the fetus, creating a connection between the sounds and the sensations.

Musical scale also has significance. Music in a minor scale will usually make us feel nostalgic or awaken memories of a sad event we experienced, as opposed to music in a joyous major scale.

Let's go back to the "Koolulam" project. Out of academic curiosity, I signed up for one of their sessions. I felt tremendous exhilaration. When all those people sang, I had a sense of friendship and togetherness. This is also biological. Shared singing causes participants to release hormones, especially oxytocin, which causes a feeling of elation.

It is similar to the feeling you will experience if you attend a service in an African-American church. Their singing is a thrilling experience that can lead to a state of meditation.

Curiously, it doesn't matter if the song is sorrowful or joyous, the important thing is that when the choir sings all together the sounds touch us and release the "good feeling" hormones.

You do not have to understand the music, simply feel it. Listening to music can be a significant tool for reducing stress, especially if we combine it with one of the other techniques outlined in the book.

Try making your lists at the end of the day accompanied by music you love. Another option is attending public singing events, mass singing such as a "Koolulam" event, or other social group singing.

Laugh Lots

Laughter is an expression of emotion. On one hand, it is an almost automatic response, but also a learned mechanism. Laughter is an expression of positive emotion for something that pleases us in the moment.

It is interesting to note that humans laugh more when they are with people than when they are alone. Laughter is often seen as a social mechanism. Laughing out loud is very easy to identify with. It is a culture-neutral mechanism, meaning that we do not know of any cultures where we are not permitted to laugh, or we do not learn to laugh.

Look at the behavior of infants who have not yet learned to speak. If you laugh at them, they will try to emulate you and test your reaction. Thus, they acquire the laughing mechanism. Tickling a baby will probably elicit sounds of pleasure and gurgling – laughter to our ears.

As adults, we have repressed the mechanism of laughter and we do not laugh very much during the day. We don't have the emotional freedom for it. Laugh at least once a day. Look for situations that make you laugh, and also try to make others laugh. In this way, you will probably also join in with their laughter as well.

Try to find the comic aspect in annoying situations. Imagine that you are a talented comedian looking for topics to laugh at for your new stand-up routine, or imagine you are a comedy sitcom writer. A comedic and entertaining perspective on everyday events will help in emotionally processing positive experiences.

Recently, an acquaintance of mine old me that in every scheduled meeting with her team at work, she tells of something that happened to her with her children or her partner and describes it so comically it makes the team members laugh. Note that laughter is an acquired mechanism, and if we do not use our ability to laugh it can wither and be lost, and that would be a shame.

Even if you are in a difficult situation, you should always try to find the humor in it and laugh at it. Often, conflict arises between conventional behavior, which is not to laugh too much, and our understanding that laughter can relieve stress or a difficulty we are experiencing.

Remember that you always feel better after a good laugh.

Nostalgic Memories

I recently was exposed to several Facebook groups with names like "childhood memories." I received lots emails and WhatsApp messages asking me if I had seen the pictures or had viewed the memories posted by childhood friends. It is interesting to note that most of us are very happy to relive these memories.

I must confess that when someone in my group uploaded a photo of classmates from elementary school, I needed help tagging some friends who have a better memory than mine. The truth is, I haven't been able to bring back negative memories from this era. One of the members put up a post asking if we remembered how we sang about love to the girls in our class.

Enjoyable, nostalgic memories enhance our current emotional state. The word nostalgia originates from the combination of "nostos" and "algos," originally from the Greek. "Nostos" means going home and "Algos" means pain. In other words, nostalgia is the pain and yearning of wanting to go home.

Nostalgia is an emotion that is not necessarily fact-based. That is why many of us tend to think that when we were children, everything was better than it is today. Nostalgia has another value that is also related to the stress issues we deal with. Nostalgia gives us a sense of warmth and allows us to feel optimistic about the future. Not only that, it can give us an empowering sense of being able to change.

Studies on the subject show that nostalgic memories and attachments enhance the way we perceive the past and the present and gives more meaning to our lives.[63]

Each of us sometimes finds himself thinking about the distant past. Sometimes our memory takes us back to a certain event. When it comes to a traumatic event, we try to understand what it was that went wrong, but also to process the feelings of pain and sorrow that memory causes us.

Sometimes, we try to think what we could have done differently. In such a situation, our imagination works overtime. We keep thinking how we would act differently or what we would say. This will usually not be easy, as we may touch the rough edges that are bare and unresolved.

Professor Constantine Sedikides, a researcher at the University of Southampton has studied the topic in collaboration with other researchers and found that compared to other memories, nostalgic memory allows us to have a positive, enjoyable, and relaxing experience.[64-65]

In the social context it is important to note that nostalgic memories can also reduce the feeling of loneliness. They allow the creation of a platform that connects people. Making contact is essential for both renewing social connections from the past and for expanding and empowering our current relationships. Nostalgic memories are also subjects for conversation, especially with those who share the same history or memories.

Sometimes, we try to think of what we would do differently. In such a situation, our imagination will work overtime. We will keep ourselves constantly thinking how we would act differently or what we would say. This will usually not be easy for us, as we may touch the edges that are bare and unresolved.

Studies also show that, like with a burst of laughter, a burst of joyful optimism is felt with nostalgic feelings. The main reason for this is that social connections make us feel a sense of higher self-esteem and this leads to a stronger sense of optimism that the future will be better (as the past was good, it is reasonable to believe that the future will also be good).[66]

Man's Search for Meaning

Can one find meaning in the most hideous and terrible situation? Viktor Frankl, in his groundbreaking book *Man's Search for Meaning*[67] teaches that even in the most horrific experience of suffering, such as that experienced by Jews during the WWII Holocaust, meaning can be found. The meaning is that living means suffering and it is man's goal to find the meaning in his suffering.

Frankl argues that there must be a purpose to life. Purpose is not universal and everyone must find his or her own purpose and meaning to life. Once we find it, we will continue to grow despite the suffering and hardships that life throws our way.

This issue has bothered me most of my adult life. What is there in life that is so important to experience? Our very existence? That is not enough.

When I asked several friends, I was surprised to learn that most of them did not understand what I was asking. They weren't bothered with wondering what the meaning of their life was, or, more precisely, they simply didn't feel the need to search for their personal purpose in this life.

I have always asked myself this question: "Suppose I died at this moment, would my life story or actions have influenced the world in any way? Or influenced the lives of others?"

I went deeper into the subject by way of self-observation, and realized that although for most of my life I have been happy and content, the question of life's meaning and purpose has affected me. I have found it exacerbated when I am in any kind of crisis, especially when there is a threat to the pleasant routine of my life (according to my interpretation, of course).

Conditions of threat to our routine can be varied and differ from one person to the next. Sometimes this happens when there is a conflict between our expectations and what happens in reality. This can manifest itself following the tragic death of a person close to us, or being fired from a job, or divorce. In these situations, the person may feel a profound sense of emptiness as a result of his suffering.

Victor Frankl suggests that each of us write a narrative of the meaning of life that suits him. Such a narrative can be expressed in giving, such as volunteering and helping others, or striving to change the world by participating in political movements, but also in a more limited way, as by focusing on one's family.

Frankl, who went through great suffering during his time in the Theresienstadt concentration camp, was able to maintain his sanity because he found meaning in his suffering. In his personal account, the very fact that he managed to retain his human spirit and the freedom to choose and still remain a good person, gave meaning to his life.

He understood that even if our time in this world is limited, and we all end our lives at some point or other (we want to believe we will live forever or at least reach a ripe old age, but no one is promised that), while we live we must find our own purpose toward which we must strive.

Frankl further added that an expectation that we will not suffer is a foolish expectation. We must understand that throughout our lives we will undoubtedly experience suffering, loss, and sorrow. Only if we have meaning in our lives, can we successfully deal with suffering and overcome it.

Sometimes, the search for meaning is in itself the purpose of our life. In the modern world of today, a working person can find meaning in his or her actions, role, or affiliation with an organization.

Professionals such as clerics, military personnel, medical personnel, police officers, firefighters, statesmen, and educators will generally sense an important purpose in their vocation. Such people are usually happier and invest their energies and purpose in their work.

Most of us seek meaning in life and repress the knowledge that one day we will cease to be. Most of our lives we won't deal with thoughts of death, otherwise anxiety will paralyze us. If we observe people with a serious illness, in many cases they will choose to fight and try to survive, despite the odds against them and despite their anxiety about death.

Finding meaning in life is an effective tool against the fear of death. I recall that once in the midst of a severe health crisis, I told my wife I would rather be an animal without consciousness and be partially happy than be a conscious, suffering person.

For me, the search for meaning is the overriding purpose in my life. One manifestation of this search for meaning is just being a father. This is a part of my life that I am very happy about. I have invested a great deal in my relationship with my children, in building relationships that are non-judgmental, respectful, and whole. I am thankful for every moment, even if it they were difficult moments, because these experiences with our family become especially significant when children arrive at the stage where they begin to search for meaning in their own lives, each in their individual way.

Various Means of Meditation

We have already dealt extensively with the importance of the daily practice of meditation. The particular method is not important, and it is even advisable to practice several methods and choose the one that works best for you. Most methods offer similar breathing and awareness techniques.

In my experience, practicing meditation in a group, especially in the early stages, can help a great deal. Search the web. There are lots of groups and sites that deal with meditation. Alternatively, you can also use an app to help you practice.

Like anything else, getting started is the hard part. It's hard to find time, because there always seems to be something more urgent. It is worthwhile to choose a regular time on your daily schedule to dedicate to meditation, preferably in the morning or the evening, but it will be fine any time during the day as well, for about ten minutes.

If you do get into the habit of practice, you will notice that after a few months there will be a significant reduction in the stress levels you are experiencing. There is no magic here, just a determination to make a change in your way of thinking and faithfully practice.

Utilizing an app also greatly enhances your skill and

commitment to daily practice. The following is a brief, but ample overview of online apps you can use for daily practice. Searching the Apple Store and Google Play Store will result in literally hundreds of options.

In this overview, I list not only some apps that I have personally tried, but also those based on a comprehensive review published in 2015, in a monthly Health Journal[68] that evaluated various apps according to functionality, visualization, information quality, exercise criteria:

- INSIGHT TIMER – Today, more than one and a half million users are registered users of this app. You will find a wide range of tools and types of meditations here. Here are some of them: Practice time periods, choosing the type of bells at the end of the sessions, and selecting the audio background. I personally choose to practice guided meditation. These are pre-recorded exercises by many instructors. Many of them are free.

- HEADSPACE – This app was established quite recently and already boasts of one famous person who uses it: actress Emma Watson. The app charges a five dollar monthly fee (the basic and first set of ten practices are free). I like this app mainly because the meditation is guided by a single instructor with an agreeable and calming voice, and is accompanied by lovely illustrations for each step. Headspace also includes a wide variety of recorded exercises on various topics such as stress reduction, reduction of anxiety, death, and more.

- SMILING MIND – This is an app and website developed by a nonprofit that aims to raise awareness for a healthier mental life. The app is free, friendly, and has over two million users including varied organizations, employers, and educators. One of the things I really like about this app is its suitability for both children and teens, and is built on defined modules and defined sessions.

- MINDFULNESS! – This is an app not only for beginners, but also for more practiced users. It offers three different guided exercises, a timer for the sessions, and meditation reminders.

- MINDFULNESS DAILY – The purpose of the app is to enable daily practice within a structured schedule. It allows you to choose a five minute daily practice session for twenty-one lessons. At the end of each session you can use the app to assess your level of stress and energy.

- 2 BUDDHIFY – a one-time paid app with a lot of content guided by various instructors. The content focuses not only on stress reduction, but also on events such as travel and hiking, waking up, taking active breaks at work, eating habits, and more. The exercises are suitable for both beginners and more experienced meditators and last between three to forty minutes, depending on your choice and level.

- AURA – This app is built in a slightly different method than the others. Each day, you will receive a new three-minute meditation practice specifically tailored for you. The app developers promise that you'll never receive the same practice more than once. Exercises can be saved for repetition as desired.

- OMVANA – This is one of the more successful apps in my opinion. OMVANA features thousands of meditations, some paid and some free. It offers beginners an eight-minute daily practice, and to the more advanced, six-step meditation is offered. The app is very similar to INSIGHTTIMER. (The more you consume the free content, the more likely you are to pay for more content.)

CHAPTER SIX

PRACTICE AND IMPLEMENTATION

"Those who have a 'why' to live, can bear with almost any 'how.'" **(Victor Frankl)**[67]

In the previous section, I elaborated on effective strategies for relieving stress. As stated, you can connect to any method you prefer. In my opinion, the most important thing is integrated training: cognitive, physical, and mental.

In this chapter, I will explain in detail how to apply the different strategies through which about change in thought patterns can be applied. If we persevere in the process, we will succeed in dealing with stress and reducing its negative impact on our lives.

Throughout my long, personal journey to discover the sources of stress and finding the tools for reducing it, I realized that knowledge was power. If we are in a crisis in our lives and are aware of our condition and the mental symptoms we are suffering from, this knowledge is of the greatest importance in our treatment and healing.

Knowledge enables us to process the steps deep into our consciousness. Slowly, and with suitable practice, we can replace bad behavior and thinking patterns with new habits and positive thought patterns that will allow us to reduce stress levels.

Practicing and applying these processes will not free us from completely having to face life's difficulties and suffering, since our emotions are of considerable importance to do so. Expecting to live a full life entirely free from suffering is impossible and will only cause us further grief. However, practice and application of meditation will reduce the intensity of stress and the length of time we suffer from anguish, which is the most important thing.

I am often asked if I have found a guaranteed recipe for success. The answer is unfortunately somewhat disappointing.

Practicing and applying the knowledge gained in this book over time will definitely improve your situation, and you will sense a significant change. But the most important thing is the decision to change your lifestyle. It's just like weight loss. If you do not change your lifestyle to a healthy, balanced one, and focus only on weighing yourself and looking at the mirror, you will probably not succeed in the long term.

The same principle applies to dealing with stress. If we make a lifestyle change and adopt a different way of thinking; following new and healthier habits, we will reduce our suffering and live better quality lives.

Now I will introduce you to a holistic training method for brain, cognitive, and physical training. There are eight rules and with daily practice you will feel a positive change in your quality of life and in your dealings with stress situations.

The holistic workout is based on daily practice at the right frequency and according to a level of intensity that changes over time. We will start with a simple, low intensity exercise and over time increase the frequency, scope, and intensity of the practice. Each exercise has a number of sets, i.e., the number of repetitions of the exercise.

Like any change that has been made in our lives, the method requires a lot of perseverance, determination, and commitment to a structured schedule. Only that way, can progress be expected. In addition, it is advisable to accompany these exercises with professionals from qualified therapists, meditation, mindfulness teachers, or life coach specialists, whichever is best for them according to their ability and preference.

Practice – Tools for Temporary Relief of Tension

This practice will help you relieve the feeling of tension almost immediately, but it does not help in the long term. The exercise is performed three times a day and involves breathing for one minute. It is an effective temporary fix when you are feeling distress, pressure, or slight anxiety.

Principle 1: Breathing Exercise

The most effective way for immediate relief from pressure is through breathing. It is desirable to practice proper breathing every day. I find myself practicing proper breathing for at least one minute five times a day. Breathing is a kind of anchor and helps us to distinguish between thought and reality.

Breathing properly trains the brain and helps lighten our burden of worrisome thoughts.

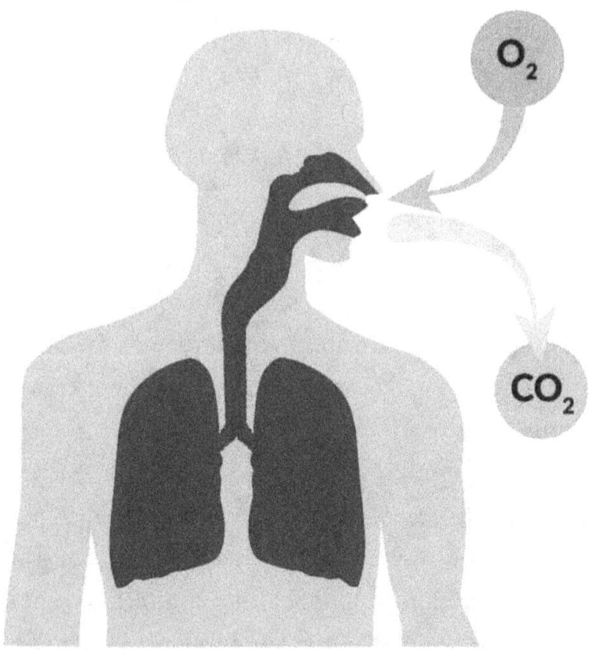

The second recommendation given here is taken from a blog published by Professor Ian Robertson.

Suppose you are an executive preparing for an important meeting, such as a meeting of the company's board of directors. Squeezing a small, soft ball in your right hand for several minutes for forty-five seconds with a fifteen-second interval between squeezes will help reduce the pressure.

Performing an action with your right hand, such as squashing the ball as we mentioned before, will awaken the left lobe of the brain responsible for a sense of challenge. As the left lobe becomes more dominant you will be able to better handle the stressful meeting.

Practice for Relief in Long-term Stress Situations

Principle 2: Meditation

Meditation is an act of introspection and non-judgmental connection between the body and the mind. There are dozens, if not hundreds of different techniques for practicing meditation, but the principle of all of them is the same: it is self-practice on a daily basis for regulating our attention and emotions.

Initially, it is important to practice with a teacher you trust, to learn to deepen the technique. You can then practice independently or use one of the effective apps available (see the previous section for a review of recommended apps).

Persistence in practice for a minimum of ten minutes a day will lead to the desired change of consciousness. I am personally very connected to the practice of mindfulness. It is a technique that incorporates ancient Buddhist principles adapted to modern life.

First Steps:

- Sit on an exercise mat, a cushion on the floor or on a comfortable chair or armchair. It's important to be relaxed and at ease.

- Close your eyes.

- Take five deep breaths (see the previous section on breathing practice).

- Breathe naturally, and as you breathe, try to imagine a large lantern light that illuminates every organ in your body. Start from the top of the head and slowly scan the rest of your body down to the tips of your fingers.

- Pay attention to your sensations and your body's contact with the floor or chair. Do you feel tension in a certain area? It's important not to want to change anything, but only be in the moment without judgment. Now go back to focusing on your breathing, is the air going out warmer than the air coming in?

- During this practice, your thoughts may wander. If that happens, merely point out to yourself that thoughts or memories are related to emotions. Do not dwell on the content. Imagine a feather stroking your thoughts and letting them continue on their way. Return your attention to the natural breathing throughout the practice as your anchor of awareness.

It is also suggested that you incorporate a personal, secular prayer or phrase that you can repeat to yourself once or twice a day. Such statements of affirmation can change your consciousness and validate what you believe in.

Some people maintain that repetition of these statements can act in a magical way and affect the mind of the believer, thus, affecting both core beliefs and the external environment.

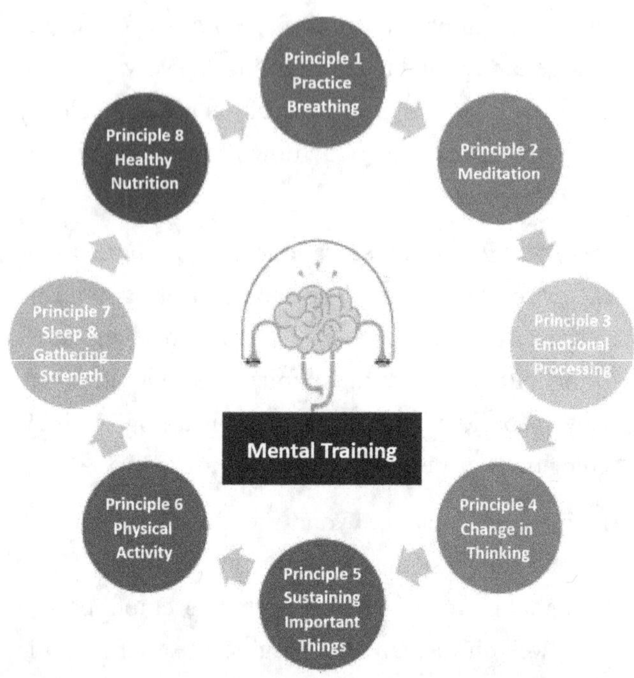

I have chosen seven statements that I repeat twice a day, in the morning and at night before bed. You are welcome to fill in the table below with your personal affirmations:

Statement/Affirmation	Content
1	
2	
3	
4	
5	
6	
7	

Principle 3: Emotions – Normalization, Ventilation, and Consolidation

Emotional processing is a tool I have found to be very effective, but like every step on this list, it also requires an appropriate method, perseverance, and connection to your emotions without fear or judgment. Emotional processing focuses on emotional thinking. That is, we need to think about the very stressors that have caused the stress we are experiencing.

As I have explained previously, many symptoms that manifest themselves in physical pain are the result of tension. In these cases, the brain chooses to deal with the feelings by diverting your attention from the emotion and creating physical pain instead. The prevention of the buildup of stress is an important day-to-day procedure that is affected by taking several actions: scanning, sorting, classifying, processing, and distribution:

Scanning

Scan all the tensions, emotions, and feelings you have had during the day. How do you do that? At the end of the day, sit down in a pleasant environment and go over the day's experiences.

I usually sit on a comfortable armchair in the bedroom, just before taking a shower. A good friend of mine does this in his car for ten minutes before heading home.

Choose a suitable time and place for yourself. After scanning, it is advisable to make a handwritten list (if you prefer to use a dedicated app or computer, that's fine too). It's a good idea to do it in table format, like the one below that I made for myself:

Personal Pressure Cooker – Month/ Day/ Year

Tension Source	Time	Physical manifes-tation	Feelings	Intensity	Details
Tax letter	Afternoon	Heart rate, gut tension	Anxiety	Medium	Feeling lasted seconds, but felt it through the day
Argument with HR manager	Morning	Felt warm, sweat, tension in chest	Anger	High	Lasted a long time, hard to calm down. Was insulted and disappointed

The Table is a tool to identify stressors and the feelings associated with them – when stress was felt and why.

Who was involved? How did it make me feel on a physical level? Sweat, fever, abdominal cramps, chest tension, lack of concentration, or emotional turmoil? How long did it last? How did it affect me during the day?

Sorting and Classification

Sorting and classification allow us to move on to the emotional processing stage. At this point, the list we have prepared, the classifications, and details, activate areas in the brain responsible for processing activity. This helps us move the data to our brain cognition area. If the list is long, it is advisable to focus on just three events that you have categorized as most intense for you.

When we recall events, it helps us understand the emotional dynamics, our reactive mechanisms, our habits, and thought patterns. In this way we prevent emotional blockage. We take some kind of "emotional shower" in addition to our regular daily shower.

Distribution and Dissemination

In the final step, it is advisable to disseminate what we have gleaned from the process. One effective way is to talk to a close friend or spouse. The very conversation and sharing allow us to vent our emotions and regularize them and feel that it was normal to react the way we did. It will also help keep things in proportion. Suddenly we won't understand why we were so upset. What was so bad?

The act of processing and classifying daily experiences in the brain will enable us to not be traumatized by the day's events. It is a good idea to consult with those close to you – friends or family – about the magnitude of the threat. Assume that a particular case was at a high level of threat, the role of your consultant is to offer you a slightly different perspective, especially on the subjective sensations you are experiencing.

Often we will use descriptive language that heightens our feelings about an event, such as, "I had a terrible day today!", "It was the worst argument I ever had.", "Nobody ever cursed at me like that!" and so on.

Separate the facts from the emotions. Don't let the

emotions unbalance your logic.

First, try to talk about the facts, and only then talk about your feelings and let your close friend or relative help you determine if the intensity of your feelings was appropriate for the situation. The important thing here is to separate feelings from fact and classify the thoughts as just "thoughts." This will greatly assist you to move from negative thoughts to positive ones and to a more optimistic perspective.

Mental Training (Principles 4-5)

Principle 4: Conceptual change – commitment, listening, skepticism, and positive commitment

Commitment results from a change in our way of thinking, which is the result of a conscious decision. Commitment to a decision and putting it into action in turn creates a process of brain training, which, like physical training, allows us to sustain what we have achieved through hard work over time.

I believe commitment and positivity are two concepts that are closely related to one another. Commitment represents a way; perseverance, determination, affection for yourself, your family, friends, and everyone around you. Positivity represents a worldview, a way we can live life.

So, should we wake up with a song in our hearts? Absolutely! We don't have to be bursting with joy and happiness, we just need to see life as being worthwhile, even if it doesn't always live up to our expectations.

Every problem has a solution, not always the solution we would have wanted at that moment, but there is a solution, and if that's the case, what is the point of worrying? Better to take things in proportion and understand that life itself strives for balance and in the medium- to long-term, everything will work out. The challenges we face are designed to teach us something about ourselves and life.

We need to ask ourselves how the challenging experience we have been through can help us gain insights that will help us in the future. Obviously not every experience is a joy, but the idea is to try to look at it from a different perspective.

Suppose you have done something offensive or dishonest, intentionally or not. And suppose only you know about it. The mere hiding and fear of discovery and its ramifications will cause you to suffer. In the short term, dealing with the problem may cause some suffering and difficulty, but it will also clear the way for stability within us by forcing us to resolve it.[1]

Often, the fear is greater than the threat itself. As we have learned, stress at some level is not necessarily a negative thing. Our brains are wired in such a way that it will be hard for us to take action if we don't even feel a little intimidated or stressed. If we feel just a little primed, our performance will only improve as long as the stress is relatively low intensity and does not last too long.

When we are feeling intimidated, look over your shoulder and if you don't see a lion striding toward you, it's likely that much of your stress is totally subjective. If that is so, your stress probably stems from ingrained thinking patterns that

---

1   "The Party's Over," music by Jule Styne, lyrics by Betty Comden and Adolph Green

have been influenced by previous events. What is important is to understand that we have control of the situation.

When you decide to commit and be positive, you must realize that this is a daily commitment. One research study found that people who daily cultivate gratitude and appreciation for what they have in life, reported better moods, a higher level of energy, and good physical health. It's worth thinking every day about something that we have experienced as positive. These can be mundane things like just getting up in the morning and feeling well.

Gratitude and Appreciation

If we query our acquaintances, we find that most of them don't really know how to answer the question, "Are you happy?"

In her book, *The How of Happiness: A New Approach to Getting the Life You Want.*[69] Dr. Sonja Lyubomirsky investigated the topic of happiness. She explains that when we talk about happiness, we have a significant bias. What is meant by that? It's that we think we know what things will make us happy and as a result we attach much greater importance to them than necessary.

Most of us think that a significant financial improvement in our lives, from a raise in salary to winning the lottery, will improve our level of happiness.

Recently, I asked a teacher what salary would make her happy. "To be realistic," she said. "An extra two thousand dollars to my salary would definitely improve my happiness quotient."

Although economic studies have found a statistical relationship between a rise in wages and an improvement in happiness,[69] money, as we know, cannot buy happiness (as long as our basic needs are met). However, our pay rise is also linked to internal reward mechanisms that make us feel satisfied (pay rise is seen as an expression of appreciation and this is what causes a rise in happiness).[69]

Suppose you receive a gift of one hundred thousand dollars. What would you do with it? In a short survey I took among family and friends, most of them mentioned material things, such as buying a car, paying off debt, and vacationing. The question is whether these are really the things that will make us happy in the long run. Personally, I am not sure.

If I am correct, there is probably no one clear recipe for happiness, but it is possible to identify ingredients that will make us feel happier, including gratitude for what we already have. An important issue in this regard is our attitude toward time. Time is an inflexible resource and we never seem to have enough of it. Be that as it may, in our daily lives we do not ask ourselves how much time we have left in this life. If we thought about that, we might well be in a constant state of panic.

We tend to repress the fact that time is a finite resource. In fact, it's rarer than diamonds. We often don't use it wisely. Let's suppose you have received a "gift" of three hours. What would you do with it? Family and friends who were asked indicated that they would fill in any gaps at work, do housework, or take the children to classes and extracurricular activities. The feeling for most of us is that we don't have enough time for everything.

Unlike money, the quantity of time is fixed and cannot be changed. In fact, the "value" of a unit of time ought to be far more significant to us than a unit of currency. It is essential that we decide what is more important to us and what is less so.

There is no secret recipe here, or rare spice that will make us happy. We need to be part of the process. Everyone needs to answer the question, "If I had more time, how would I utilize it to increase the level of happiness in my life?"

Psychologist Dan Gilbert in his book, *Stumbling on Happiness*,[70] demonstrates through arguments based on many studies how one can achieve a feeling of happiness.

If you ask people what they think about the majority of the time, the past, present, or future, you will find that most will say they think about the future. Research on the subject found that in the stream of consciousness, an average 12 percent of our daily thoughts are on the future.[70] Why is this so? Why can't we just be in the here and now?

Exercises:

1. Make a note of the things in your life that are important to you and make you feel good. Do it every day! Try to write down at least one new thing every day.

2. Write down several ways you can invest small amounts of money for services that will save you time and give you pleasure. Maybe, once a month, spend fifty dollars for a babysitter and go out for a meal with your spouse. You can also hire a house cleaner and use the time you are free to go to the beach and enjoy the sunset, etc.

3. Be in "tune" with yourself every day for at least half an hour instead of being busy with regular tasks. Try sitting in a cafe alone, or read a book, or listen to music, sit on the porch and people watch, etc.

Most of us don't really listen to ourselves or to those around us. Most of the time we judge ourselves by a list of things that "need to be done." This list, by the way, will fill up almost nonstop, no matter how many things we cross off as having already done them.

Practice 1:

Take a pen and paper and list, without any order of importance, everything you think you need to do. Write it all down. Work issues, home, family, relationships, money, trips, shopping, and anything else that comes to mind. Now, underline or mark everything you can't give up and must do. When you are done, turn the page over.

Now write down your inventory, meaning your resources, either tangible or intangible. Let your mind randomly search and write down everything that comes to mind: home, family, friends, work, and experiences. List as much as possible and be specific.

My list consisted of my mother Rachel, Grandma Veronica, electric guitar, a house with a garden, a vintage living room, etc. Now on your list underline the things that would never part with and what you value as most important to you.

Look at the two lists and ask yourself, "What is your

conclusion? What is shaping me and has formulated my life? What feelings did I have for what I wrote on each of the lists? What would I like to change and what recurrent pattern do I see?"

This practice will help you carry out a self-observation process. This way you can understand the connection between what you want and what really matters.

Practice 2:

It is worthwhile finding time during our busy daily schedule for what we call "a quiet island." It is recommended that we make time between work meetings. Even five minutes will suffice. In addition, in the afternoon you should also allocate a few minutes to "abstaining from email and the phone," where you will not call or send messages, but simply make time for yourself.

At first it will be a little difficult, but over time you will feel that you need this time. These moments are important, they soothe the nervous system, conserve energy, and develop our mental capacity.

Listening to ourselves is important, but how much do we really listen to others? When we speak to someone, we spend a great deal of time thinking about what we want to say next, not really what we are hearing.

Or, we reflect on what we have to do today, what things at home or at work haven't I done yet? What we learn from this is that we actually spend only a small fraction of our time really listening. It is important that we practice active listening. Here are a few simple techniques for you:

Active Listening Practice:

During a meeting, write down important points that come up in the conversation. Use the mirroring technique, such as "You say we should invest more money in accessing the services." That is a mirroring operation. Now address the issue and respond accordingly, "This is an important point. I would like more details on it from you so we can make a decision later."

With active listening, we allow the brain to rest and focus energy on what is happening right now, and not allow our thoughts to wander. The goal of the practice is on one hand, to reduce the waste of energy and preserve it over time, and in the same manner improve our mental capacity.

Doubts

So as to not get bogged down in negative thoughts, it is advisable to practice a way of thinking that will help us see things in proportion. It is important for our thoughts to be commensurate with their true weight in the reality of our lives.

Practice:

When a thought comes to mind, write it down. Now go into detail: What are the facts the thought is based on? Is it repetitive? How much control do we have over the thought? What are the chances of it being realized or not?

The thought	Support points	Opposing points	Recurring or new	Chances it will happen	Doubts
I am going to be fired	Manager makes a sour face. My request for promotion denied	My colleagues value me. I meet my goals. I am dedicated to my job	Thought recurs appx once a week	50-50	My interpretation. A fairly good chance it won't happen

Meaning

We all need meaning in our lives. In order to attain a personal meaning for ourselves, we should ask the question, "Why? Why do we do the work we do? Why are we in the relationship we are in? Why do we react the way we do in stressful situations?" If we ask ourselves these questions, we have to provide answers, and this will require us to really consider and search for reasons for the things we do and think.

Practice

Take a paper and pen and next to each question and answer, write down three positive details and three less than positive ones.

I wrote: Why do I work in the job I now have? Answer: Because the company is a leader in the field, and I have a family to support.

- Three positives: decent salary, job satisfaction, convenient working hours.
- Three negatives: No promotion options, the field is not of great interest to me, lots of pressure at work.

Keep practicing and write down the things you like to do and why you like doing them. This is an important question.

Thomas S. Monson, a former head of the Church of the Latter Day Saints once said, "Choose your love, love your choice." Meaning that once you understand what you really love, choose to do it and teach yourself to love it even more.

Happiness, as we know, is not for sale in a store, it must stem only from our understanding that we are happy, and not from a stack of commodities and groceries.

At the end of the process I have outlined you will be better able to understand what your meaning or purpose in life is. Your purpose does not have to be something as earth-shattering as "repairing the world," or correcting the ills in our country, causing happiness for another by giving, helping others, and empowering others. It can be simpler things such as building a family, child rearing, personal development, or friendships.

Principle 5: Preserve what is important in social and family relationships.

From my childhood I was taught that family is the most important part of our lives. Is it really? It depends, of course, on who you ask and which family you belong to.

When I speak of family, I do not necessarily mean a

biological family, but one that we define as our family. Members of this family can be close or distant relatives, but they can also be friends from childhood, work, the military, or any other circle. The formulation is personal and is determined by the level of trust and intimacy among the members of the group you define as family.

People close to us are very important in our lives. In the process of change, relatives are of even greater significance because in such a time we need a supportive, loving, and mostly non-judgmental environment.

Remember that relationships need maintenance, preservation, and nurturing, so invest time and thought into each relationship the best you can. The essential principle in relationships with people is to try not to be judgmental; not of others, and of yourself.

For example, if in the near future my personal priorities require a greater investment of time in others and as a result I will see less of my parents, it is best to understand and accept the situation. It is not desirable to judge myself severely and think I am neglecting my parents or failing to meet my expectations. I will reflect on the situation with those closest to me and, in most cases, they will understand it.

It is useful to make a list of things that are important to me in the coming weeks. The list must be realistic. If it is not feasible to visit elderly parents twice a week but only once in two weeks, do so and speak to them by phone the other times.

It is important to include in social and family relationships the people who are good for you and pleasant to be with. Try not to include those you are not good with, even if your social circle expects you to. If it is difficult to avoid contact with these people, you can simply reduce the frequency and duration of your meetings.

Close relationships with the people we care about can be helpful and supportive. In addition, maintaining a nurturing relationship with those close to us is essential to the emotional regulation we undergo when dealing with the stresses in our lives.

Practice:

Make a list of the ten most important people in your life (or less, if you don't have ten).

Outline the frequency of meetings and conversations for the coming week. Take into account that there may be changes. What matters is the intent and not necessarily the implementation. If you fail to make all the meetings you wanted to, it's not a catastrophe. You can always talk on the phone or correspond by messages on your smartphone.

Work

For most of us, work plays a central role in our lives. It is not only the economic aspect that is the most important thing, but also stability and personal development. In addition, research shows that people who work and are busy live longer and, in particular, healthier lives.

Work is a source of livelihood, but sometimes it is also an ongoing source of stress. Many of those around me tell me how much they are waiting when they can afford to stop working and spend their time leisurely studying and traveling. I personally disagree with this goal and think it is essential to continue working. Sometimes it is possible to adjust the quantity and scope of your work, but work is important as it enables us to face constant challenges.

Work also provides us a modicum of stress that allows the brain to remain vital and to continue to develop, even into old age. Also, work helps us to preserve memory. It is important to understand that even if work is at the top of our list of stressors, much of its effects depend on us, regulated by our approach to stress, and degree of flexibility.

One of the most common concepts today in the world of work is work resilience, i.e., our capacity (which can, of course, be developed and nurtured) to absorb and cope with change and challenges in the workplace.

A practice that helps increase work resilience will include an effective agenda for active work breaks. A concept that has taken root in this context is "workplace agility," which refers to the relationship between liveliness and flexibility.

Practice:

Set up an efficient schedule – Research shows that a carefully formulated agenda, but one that also has the flexibility for change, will help reduce cognitive overload. Embed a list of tasks of the same type into a predefined time window and do nothing else in that same window.

Such as, between eight and nine in the morning reply to emails. During this period do not answer phone calls (unless they are from very important sources that you have categorized in advance) or WhatsApp messages, do not read anything and do not authorize invoices.

Despite what is commonly thought, it is more important to effectively manage a single-task rather than multi-task.

Shawn Achor, in his best-selling book *The Happiness Advantage*,[71] lists seven ways in which positive psychology will help us improve performance and success in the workplace.

It turns out that every minute of our work lives, we absorb about eleven million bits of information, but our brains are capable of processing only 40 percent of that amount in one minute.[71]

Compiling tasks at work and dividing them into similar categories will allow us to manage them more effectively and reduce our cognitive load.[71]

Mental availability – The concepts of agility and flexibility are from the world of physical education, but they are also suitable for the mental environment. The main point is that when we are in a state of stress we can be able to pause for a moment, sit back, reflect, change our perspective, create new choices, and choose wisely.[72]

In this practice, when we pause for a moment and reflect on the problem we are facing, we shift our focus to the more conscious and analytical parts than the emotional ones. This technique will allow us, over time, to improve coping with stress and to nurture our cognitive ability.

Compassion and Judgment – Compassion for ourselves and those around allows us to foster positive emotions and improve relationships with our colleagues and superiors.

For example, if your colleague looks a little scruffy today and is possibly angry and upset, try to understand the factors that led to it and show compassion.

Compassion also helps reduce judgment and ultimately enables a supportive and balanced relationship between colleagues in the workplace.

A report by the multinational professional services network PricewaterhouseCoopers – PWC,[73] found that the Return on Investment Index (ROI) was 2.3, which means that every dollar spent on programs to increase cognitive flexibility in the workplace saved about 2.3 dollars as a result of reducing absenteeism and increasing effectiveness.

Sources of Inspiration Through Mentoring

A mentor (from Greek) is a person who serves as a consultant or guide. In Greek mythology, Mentor was the friend of Odysseus, who in turn served as a mentor to his son Telemachus.

The word mentor represents a person with rich experience in his or her field of business or in life, who can act as a guide or advisor to a young person or alternatively to anyone who needs guidance.

Today, the phenomenon of mentoring is widely accepted in the business and academic worlds, but it is also common among large organizations that have institutionalized mentoring initiation processes within their enterprises. Research has proven that mentoring is important in the workplace and has a positive effect on reducing employee burnout.

A 2014 study[74] found that mentoring can reduce the intensity of stress a person experiences in their workplace. The mentor provides the person with whom he or she works with both psychological support as well as counseling and guidance. The mentor is a personal example and serves as a source of inspiration, affirmation, and the presentation of a variety of perspectives.

Imagine a situation (which many of you have encountered) in which you sent a personal request by email to your manager and did not receive a response. Several days go by and the manager still has not responded. If you have a tendency toward neuroticism, your thoughts are likely to continually trouble you, "Why didn't I get an answer? Is it because the answer is no?"

The anticipation and disappointment can also be expressed in anger, "Who does he think he is? Why doesn't he answer, or at least confirm that he received the email?" In such a case, a mentor can certainly help to enable the employee to view the situation from a different perspective, as well as listen to and support the employee's feelings.

The mentor will reflect on the situation and reassure him and possibly tell him that they were in such a situation in the past as well, and that chances are he did not return the email due to technical matters or time constraints. In this way, the mentor helps the employee conceive of a logical answer that will divert his negative thoughts.

A mentor's feedback and attitude are seen as valid; they can calm us down and reduce burnout in the workplace. The mentor can also affect our private lives. It is important to note that a good mentor is one with whom we can establish a trusting relationship, so we can talk with transparency and openness. The role of the mentor is primarily to assist us in the social and psychological aspects of our lives and less in the managerial or business aspects.

Interaction with the mentor usually occurs in face-to-face meetings but learning processes from other sources of inspiration can also help. If we do a process of reflection and projection of other people's stories into our own lives, it can help us with the self-observation that each of us must do. This is another tool in our toolkit that can help regulate the effects of stress on our lives.

Practice:

1. Go over your list of acquaintances and try to identify someone you connect with easily who has rich life experience. Contact him or her and find out if they would be willing to be your mentor.

2. If this is not feasible, you can hire mentoring services from one of the leading companies in the field. Go to Google, you will find many recommendations.

3. Look for people you identify with and who inspire you. Learn their personal stories, make a list of insights about your life from what you have read and learned. Try to incorporate them into your own life and decide which of the insights you have accumulated to utilize, and when.

Physical Exercise (Principles 6-8):

Physical exercise training is the third part of the program I have outlined in this chapter. There are three inseparable components: exercise, sleep, and proper nutrition.

Principle 6: Exercise

Physical exercise is vital and has an impact on many aspects of our lives. A person who is physically active will improve his health and, most probably, his sense of well-being.

What does it mean to be physically active? What kind of exercise? What is the frequency, intensity, amount of exercise necessary?

The short answer is that it doesn't matter what you do, the main thing is to be active. The more thorough answer is that it is desirable to do moderate exercise, one that is professionally guided and tailored to your abilities. Optimal exercise is one that is graded by level and performed regularly on a daily and weekly basis.

On a daily basis, the aim is to adopt an active lifestyle, such as walking or riding a bicycle instead of using a motorized vehicle, and preferring to climb stairs rather than take an elevator, etc. Exercise affects the condition of our heart and lungs as well as the skeletal and muscular system.

Research also shows that exercise positively affects learning, memory, and other cognitive functions, because physical activity increases oxygen consumption as well as the level of neurotransmitters (such as serotonin and norepinephrine) in the regions of the brain that are essential in the performance of tasks.[75]

In addition, many studies have shown that physical activity is directly related to the regulation of stress. Unfortunately, only a relatively small percentage of the population in the Western world is regularly active.

The reasons for this are varied, from claims of lack of time to low self-esteem, economic considerations, and difficulty in commitment, dedication, discipline, and more. Most of us just aren't interested. It is easier to keep smoking, consuming alcohol, and eating whatever comes our way, even though we are aware of the many benefits of exercise.

Why is exercise so stress-related? Our brain interprets physical activity as a state of stress. Think about it, the characteristics are similar: increased pulse rate, sweat, increased activity of the skeletal system and muscles. All of this is compatible with stress and threat, but in the case of exercise the brain makes the event a positive one and that allows us to improve our capability for less investment of energy.

A person who regularly exercises can easily switch between stress and relaxation states. Also, when performing intense physical activities such as running, dancing, kickboxing, etc., the brain has no chance to engage in troubling everyday thoughts and instead, is entirely centered on the physical activity. You could say this is a kind of "active" meditation.

The brain is the central element that affects both our physical and our mental states. Accordingly, one of the main propositions in this book is that there is no difference between body and mind. The point is to be physically active, no matter how.

I personally recommend combining physical activity with either walking or running and yoga. When we exercise, such as running or strength training, we significantly increase our blood flow rate and that, in and of itself, improves brain performance.

In his book, *The Spark*, psychiatrist John Ratey[76] explains that running and strength training not only improve performance, but also combat stress, anxiety, depression, addiction, and even slow down the aging of brain cells.

According to Ratey, this contributes to the balance of neurotransmitters (such as serotonin, norepinephrine, and dopamine) and battles chronic stress in which there is a deletion of nerve cell connections or a contraction of certain areas of the brain.

Exercise allows the brain to stimulate learning, adapting to different situations and improving thinking processes.[76] It creates a balance between the different systems in the brain. Physical activity improves brain function, and in this way the brain can better cope with stress.[76]

In fact, the brain responds to activity just as muscles respond to exercise. Regular exercise produces proteins in the body that circulate in the bloodstream and reach the brain. Physical exercise has a huge impact on cognitive, health, and mental abilities.

What is yoga and why is it important?

Yoga is a physical activity derived from Hindu culture. It combines physical and spiritual training and perceives them as a single entity. Yoga has existed for thousands of years in many incarnations and developments. Yoga practice has significant physical benefits, such as improving muscle flexibility and strength, but it is also a spiritual journey toward consciousness. The practice of yoga allows the practitioner to acquire spiritual tools for dealing with life's difficulties.

Yoga is based on the practice of "asana" (the Sanskrit word means "to be in a certain state"). Asanas are postures that have evolved over many years, each concentrating on certain areas and systems in the body. Yoga helps the body to develop, to be stable, strong, flexible, and like mindfulness, it also incorporates breathing awareness, listening to the body, and movement repetition that focuses the mind on exercise rather than on daily thoughts and reflections.

Although there are various techniques for yoga practice, the basis of yoga is the same. That is, a sequence of postures aimed at strengthening the muscles and improving the flexibility of the joints. As in meditation, breathing also plays an important part in yoga. The control of breath is the beginning of the control of consciousness.

In a 2015 report, one of the most famous hospitals in the United States found that yoga had a major impact on coping with stress. Studies have also shown improvements in various health measures in people who regularly practice yoga.[29]

Yoga is suitable for everyone. There is no age or fitness limit. Beginner practice requires a proper guide and perseverance, learning postures, listening to the body, and progressing in a steady manner. All of these steps will strengthen the muscles, improve flexibility, increase stability, and build up your balance, but also enhance the mind-body connection.

Start out with a steady, graded level of guided exercise at least three times a week, for an hour. There is another option: "run, walk, run" that has gained momentum in recent years and is based on a mix of running and walking.

The method was originally developed by Jeff Galloway, a sprinter who ran competitive middle-distance races. At present, three hundred thousand runners practice this method around the world, and teams from eighty cities in the United States and five countries outside the U.S., have developed their abilities the most.

This method is based on taking small steps close to the ground and interrupting the running sequence with walks. The running is timed minute by minute and progresses to five minutes running and one minute of walking. Do not run for more than six consecutive minutes to prevent injuries. For more information, visit Jeff Galloway's website.

Practice:

1. It is recommended to use one or the other method (in a progressive manner and after a checkup by your family doctor) at least twice a week, and practice yoga at least twice a week.

2. As you progress, you can increase the frequency and duration of the activity. Please note that over-training can lead to injury and long-term damage.

Principle 7: Sleep and the Power nap

Strange as it may sound, sleep is a great tool for dealing with stress. When we are stressed, we are in a vicious negative cycle. When we are very disturbed (especially stress is chronic), our thoughts also intrude into our minds at night and we can find it hard to fall asleep. Due to a lack of sleep we become more tired and the accumulated fatigue makes it difficult for us to cope well with stress and its recurrence.

The recommendation that is repeated in almost all studies in the field is to go to sleep at a regular time for a full eight hours a night. A nap in the afternoon, the "powernap" is also important.

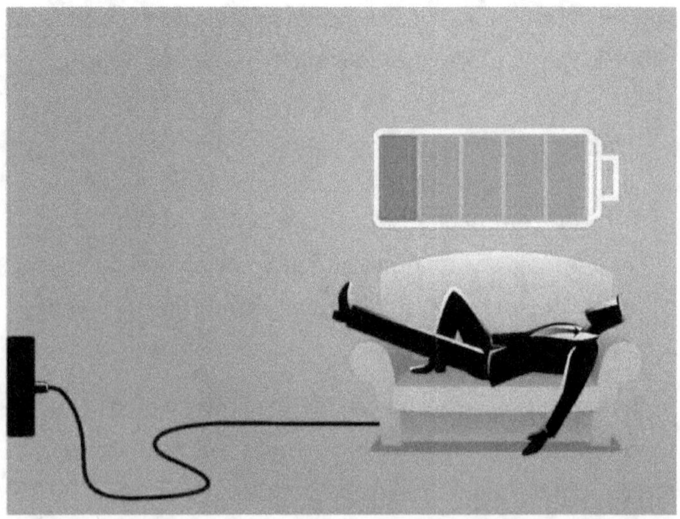

The powernap is short-term day time sleep (rather than in the evening hours) of about twenty minutes on average. Longer durations will lead to the sleep onset state (R.E.M.)

that is not desirable during day time.

Studies have shown that workers who take a powernap during the day show great improvement in productivity. The improvement is evident in aspects such as creativity, visual perception, information processing, and associative thinking.[77] Such sleep also improves alertness.

I especially recommend the powernap for managers whose schedule is packed with numerous meetings and phone calls.

There are countries where this is an established way of life: In Spain it is the Siesta, in Italy the Riposo, and in the United States, companies that give time and thought to improving the quality of the lives of their employee, have set up areas designated for powernaps and meditation.

Practice:

1. Seating – If there is no comfortable bed or sofa available, you can doze off seated in a comfortable armchair. Your legs should be elevated, and it is desirable to use a comfortable pillow for your back and head that can be kept in the office for this purpose.

2. Turn off phones and computers – Earplugs will help muffle sound. Darken the room, but not completely. If it is difficult to make the room dark, you can use an eye mask made of healthy material. If you are not an earplug enthusiast, there are high-quality headphones that isolate external noises.

3. Quiet time – Some people prefer complete silence,

but others prefer "white noise." Specific sound frequency can be chosen with dedicated apps (download a "white noise" app from your iPhone or Android smartphone).

4. Temperature – Studies have shown that the optimum temperature for sleep is a cool sixty-two to sixty-six degrees Fahrenheit or seventeen to nineteen degrees Celsius, so it is advisable to cover yourself with a light blanket.

5. Routine – Set a regular time for this light sleep during the day. It is highly desirable to have it after lunch, but be careful not to consume caffeine, sugar, fat-saturated foods, or sugary drinks at least an hour before the nap.

6. Apps – There are quite a few apps that help with sleep: SLEEPSMART, a pleasant, free app that has options for playing a "white noise" sound, setting an alarm, as well as Relax Melodies. Google has a vast selection to check out.

As for guilt feelings – forget about them! Thoughts such as, "If I doze off in the middle of the day, I'm lazy," should be replaced by, "I'm so busy that the nap will give me the strength and energy to continue," or, "A nap is important for my quality of life."

Like everything else in life, we are often required to adapt to a different lifestyle than we are used to. It is important to understand that change, in the beginning, will not be easy and that we need discipline, determination, and perseverance.

Principle 8: Proper Nutrition

What has an effect on what? Does nutrition affect mood or does mood affect nutrition? There is probably no definitive answer to this question. Dietitians and physicians recommend proper nutrition: avoiding or reducing the intake of caffeinated beverages (coffee, tea, cocoa, chocolate, or cola). These create a temporary feeling of alertness that will soon be replaced by fatigue and stress.

It is also not recommended to consume products such as spices, fried foods, fats, or even simple sugars (such as in sweetened foods). They are not recommended as they cause an imbalance in blood sugar and may increase the tendency to be vulnerable to stress. The same goes for protein intake. Protein stimulates the nervous system in the body. On one hand, it makes us more alert, but too much animal protein can cause restlessness and tension. Alcohol and nicotine intake are also not recommended.

Meat, and especially fatty meat, also increases the feeling of tension and anxiety. Eating meat causes the release of dopamine, which taxes the blood vessels and the heart.

Chemicals present in processed foods, such as preservatives and artificial flavors and scents, are a burden on the liver, which is the organ responsible for filtering out toxins in the body, which in turn, affects overall mood.

If all these foods are harmful, how can nutrition reduce stress?

It turns out it is possible. Experts say a carbohydrate-rich menu will increase the secretion of serotonin in the brain and raise the sense of calm and relaxation. Serotonin is a neurotransmitter; a molecule that passes between a nerve cell (neuron) and a target cell through the synapse. Serotonin relaxes, improves mood, and contributes to a feeling of satiety. When our blood level is high in serotonin, we are calm, and when it is low we feel nervous and impatient.

Complex carbohydrates are preferable over simple carbohydrates. Complex carbohydrates are found in rice, potatoes, buckwheat, quinoa, wheat, oats, and whole grains. They take longer to digest than simple carbohydrates such as corn syrup, sugar, etc.

Magnesium-rich foods are also recommended during periods of stress. Low magnesium levels are known to cause symptoms, such as headaches and fatigue, which can exacerbate stress.

Green vegetables such as spinach, broccoli, celery, mangold, flax seeds, pumpkin seeds, and sunflowers are rich in magnesium. Green vegetables are highly recommended. They are rich in folic acid, which participates in the production of dopamine – another neurotransmitter that allows us to feel happiness, pleasure, vigor, motivation, focus, and concentration. A combination of multi-colored vegetables as part of your daily menu will give your body the vitamins, minerals, and antioxidants that it needs, especially in times of stress.

Dark chocolate, which contains magnesium, is another recommendation. Studies have shown that cortisol levels (the stress hormone) in people who eat up to a quarter cup or twenty grams of dark chocolate daily for two weeks were low compared to those who ate a different snack food in the same amount. Remember, however, that chocolate has lots of fat and is high in calories, so it is important not to overdo it. Dark chocolate containing at least 60 percent cocoa solids is preferable.

It is also recommended to consume fatty acids from the Omega-3 family. Linolenic is an essential fatty acid which must be obtained from food, as the body cannot produce it on its own. From Omega-3, the body creates an enzymatic process chain which produces a number of important fatty acids, including DHA EPAA. These fatty acids have anti-inflammatory properties that can combat the negative effects of stress hormones. DHA is critical for brain cell structure, and EPA helps neuron function and even reduces inflammation.

Studies have shown that acids also contribute to alleviating depression and anxiety. Omega-3 is found mainly in salmon, tuna, mullet, trout, flax seeds, and walnuts. The recommendation is to consume fish at least twice a week. To increase the effect, you can take a concentrated food supplement of Omega-3 and escalate its influence on mood.

I recently went to a high quality restaurant and had a good meal. After I finished it, I said I was "stuffed" and had no room for anything more. But then came the dessert menu and it featured a cheesecake that I love. I decided to order it, even though at the moment I felt "stuffed" and had declared that I couldn't eat another thing for the next few hours.

Why was this happening? Why is it that even though my stomach was full, I still found room for delicious cheesecake? The answer is the brain. The brain determined my stuffed feeling wasn't so bad; there was more room in my stomach. The sweetness of the dessert is the reward the brain has as its aim. The photo on the menu and the words "cheesecake" stimulated a part of the brain that recalled the enjoyable feeling of eating cheesecake and decided it wanted its reward.

We eat "with our eyes," and with the memories and sensations that food has left us with. We also eat according to the habits we have established over the years. Our minds like patterns, both bad and good. If we don't teach the brain what is good for us and what is bad, the brain will make the same decisions it is used to making because it does not require it to expend any energy. In this way, the automatic cognitive patterns will dictate our behavior.

So, I ordered my cheesecake, although I really didn't need it, neither nutritionally nor to feel better. The brain, among other things, manages the balance of energy in the body, so when we feel weak, off balance, or emotionally fragile, the brain will search for an available source of light energy for us and what is simpler than food for the soul?

The brain was looking for available energy and we created a cycle of punishment and pleasure related to eating, and especially to emotional eating.

A study by a group of researchers at the University of California in 2007, dealt with exactly this reward mechanism. They found that stress and emotional eating mechanisms are closely related.[73]

The combination of stress and eating, what we perceive to be tasty, produces an internal opioid release. This opioid release is also linked to the brain's defense mechanism against stress. Augmented exposure to one of two conditions: stress or eating food that pleases us, can lead to improper habits for emotional needs.[78]

CONCLUSION

There are few occasions in life when a person can say that they have changed. Most of us do not change.

As it was written on the gravestone of Swiss mathematician Jacques Bernoulli: "Although (I have) changed, I rise again (remain) the same."

Following on Bernoulli's epitaph, I can personally testify that I have been able to change negative thinking patterns through intensive daily practice. I have changed the way I conduct my life, but I have retained my values and my essence that are the foundations of my personality.

Sometimes I do find myself worrying or feeling agitated, but I can thankfully say that I have learned to differentiate between real threat situations and unsubstantiated worries. Worries may possibly become real threats, but the emphasis is that this is only a possibility, not reality.

Through regular practice the brain learns and alters its responses. If you haven't absorbed it by now, remember we will all die in the end; the question is how we live our lives until then. I have chosen to look at my time on earth as a gift that I must cherish, honor, and live as best I can.

Time is one of the recurring motifs in this book, interwoven throughout. Time, unlike many other things in life, is a constant. There are only twenty-four hours in a day, period.

The question I asked myself when I began my research and started writing down my thoughts was how should I live my life in my limited time on this earth?

I am reminded of the immortal words of Ecclesiastes, chapter three: "There is a time for everything, and a season for every activity under the heavens." And I wondered, was Ecclesiastes, right? Is there is a time for everything?

After turning this question around in my mind, I came across the work of the famous poet Yehuda Amichai, *A Man in His Life*,[79] who attempts to debate this statement of Ecclesiastes.

My conclusion from reading this work is that life happens in the here and now and not in our thoughts. Our thoughts play an important role in our lives, but our thinking does not really have the power to change reality, only the power to influence our behavior and the actions we take.

Throughout our lives we will experience events that our brains classify as threats and which will greatly affect our quality of life. Stress is definitely a product of how we interpret the events around us and especially those events that pertain to us personally.

As long as the power and frequency of stress are in the right dosages, its effect will be limited and even provide us with the motivation to improve. However, long-lasting, high-intensity stress can lead to mental illnesses such as anxiety disorders, clinical depression, and physical illnesses such as heart disease, cancer, and chronic pain.

All of us can deal with stress; all it takes is knowledge, awareness, and perseverance in implementing an appropriate lifestyle. Coping with stress is possible and it will help us over time to have the flexibility to adapt our behavior and recover from stressful situations. This capability can be learned.

Studies in the field have shown that when we develop the ability to recover and cope, traumatic conditions such as near-death events can be recovered from quite quickly.[80]

There is no one best strategy for everyone. Each person must find the tools to help them develop these capabilities. In the previous chapter, I suggested several ways that have proved successful. Each of us must adopt strategies that allow to replace old habits and thinking patterns with newer, more successful ones: by processing and venting our feelings, sharing with others, and by exercising, our brain will develop coping and recovery skills.

People who have developed this ability will be able to read situations accurately and find the appropriate response to the situation. They will be able to choose from a variety of response modes they have adopted for themselves and that are working for them. This is called "recalibration."

The ability to "re-calibrate" or "restart" is usually innate, but we can all develop it further. Psychologists even argue that it is important and essential that children be exposed to difficulties, failures, and allowed to make mistakes at an early age.

I remember vividly how I watched a once admired relative who, until a relatively mature age, succeeded in everything he touched: his studies, work, and personal life. Without going into an in-depth discussion about what success actually is, when that relative experienced a business failure for the first time in his life, and as a result his marriage also fell apart, he collapsed for a long time, and only through intensive therapy was he able to return to some kind of a stable routine.

Dealing with difficulties previously would have helped him recover faster from the setbacks he experienced. The opposite situation, where only failure has been experienced, is also undesirable.

We need to experience everything in life, but in the required doses. It is important for us to find at least one good trait in each of our children, and to help that child feel a sense of success that is so important to mental health.

When we deal with a problem, failure, or any situation that we have classified as threatening, over-engaging in the problem or cause of stress will only exacerbate the suffering. Over-engaging is usually done through rumination and immersion in the negative thoughts related to the problem we are currently dealing with.

Of course, our personality also has an impact on our ability to cope. Neurotic types have a higher tendency to suffer from stress due to a negative view of possible outcomes. When a person's perception of reality is negative, it is difficult to develop mechanisms and tools for coping with even healthy and flexible stressors. By contrast, people with self-awareness of their abilities, skills, and who have high self-esteem tend to cope better with stressful situations.

The important thing is not whether you have the ability to cope, but whether you believe you do. As we saw in the very first chapter of this book, the brain is flexible and the way we think and choose to act will have a definite impact on how it functions.

The bottom line is we all face situations of stress of some kind or other. Such situations cannot be prevented or avoided completely (in fact, avoidance can have the opposite effect and make the problem worse). If we realize that unpleasant events are an integral part of life and adopt coping strategies that enable us to gain more effective thinking and behavior patterns, we can overcome the difficulties and take control of our lives.

Linda Graham in the introduction to her book, *Bouncing Back: Rewiring Your Brain for Maximum Resilience and Well-Being*,[70] demonstrates how five processes each of us adopt will enable the development of coping skills and recovery from stress.

She calls them, "The five Cs of resilient coping." They are:

1. Calm – You can stay calm in a crisis.

2. Clarity – You can see clearly what's happening as well as your internal response to what's happening; you can see what needs to happen next; and you can see possibilities from different perspectives that will enhance your ability to respond flexibly.

3. Connection – You can reach out for help as needed; you can learn from others how to be resilient; and you can connect to resources that greatly expand your options.

4. Competence – You can call on skills and competencies that you have learned through previous experience (or that you learn) to act quickly and effectively.

5. Courage – You can strengthen your faith to persevere in your actions until you come to resolution or acceptance of the difficulty.

Changing thinking, or more accurately balancing new patterns and ways of thinking, is an important element in the stress regulation process, as well as being able to cope with stress when it comes back. It is important to remember that the brain, due to its law of energy conservation, prefers set patterns, and does not prioritize randomness.[81]

Two additional factors are social learning and associative learning. Dean Burnett in his book, *The Idiot Brain*[81] explains how the brain is affected by both of these.

Social learning is learning from the actions of others either by observing them or imitating best practices. In the context of stress, it is about observing how others respond to stress and threat situations and imitate the way they cope with it.

Burnett offers an example by citing a study in which chimpanzees learned to be afraid of snakes. They were not afraid because they feared attack, but because they observed others who were afraid and so they learned to fear themselves. The brain adapts a pattern of behavior influenced by watching others' reactions to the same stressful situation.

We also learn by association, but Burnett argues that we can get rid of patterns that have taken root in our minds. It calls this extinction, which means that we have to teach the brain that a particular stimulus does not necessarily have to be met with our habitual reaction. Therefore, the brain's accustomed response to the stimulus is unnecessary.

For example, if a regularly scheduled meeting with your manager creates anxiety in you, then a number of these sessions that end without a negative result, will enable you to extinguish the habit of perceiving the meetings with the negative association you had been accustomed to.

Patterns created on the basis of negative past events affect our biological system, including cell development. Studies in a relatively new field called epigenetics have found that cells are influenced mainly by the interconnection they have with the environment. This statement is contrary to the popular notion that the genetic code, our DNA, is the determining factor. In fact, some think that, as they are a particular type of energy, thoughts have a direct effect on the function of protein production in cells.

In his fascinating book, *The Biology of Faith*[82] developmental biologist Dr. Bruce Lipton describes how a particular perception or belief creates reality and influences how our body grows or ceases its biological growth.

He argues that from a psychological perspective, when we react to a stressful situation, the brain prefers that all accessible energy will be invested in allowing us to escape as quickly as we can from a situation we have identified as dangerous.

When we remain for a long period in a stressful state, growth ability is inhibited because our blood supply is concentrated only on the vital organs, we need to be able to escape. Harnessing all the physical energy in order to deal with a threat also causes the immune system to be muted.

Lipton illustrates this phenomenon visually: "Let's say we are ill with a virus and suddenly come across a roaring lion facing us. The brain, first, will deal with the immediate threat, i.e., the roaring lion (analogous to stress) and reduce the energy directed to the immune system for fighting the virus."

In this automated system, the lion is the immediate

danger and not the virus. In such a situation, both the speed of thinking and our ability to analyze are impaired, as the energy in the brain is directed solely to processing the information necessary for our physical survival.

These automatic mechanisms are essential for survival in a real threat situation. In modern life, we need to train the mind to distinguish between actual physical threats and worrying thoughts or moments of stress. Most of the pressures we face do not pose a physical danger to our existence.

In fact, our brain is over-active. Not only that, some of us have embedded in our brains an unrealistic thinking pattern, that is, a brain pattern that focuses on possible negative consequences of events that have not yet happened[81] but we classify them as potential threats.

Suppose I am invited to a conference with a large number of participants. A few days before the event, I already feel distressed, my mouth is dry, I feel weak, and have no desire to take part in activities such as sports or seeing friends. The brain has classified the upcoming event as negative, even though it has not yet taken place.

An excellent tool to train the brain to adopt a different thinking pattern is to attend the meeting and at the conclusion, even if it was partially unpleasant, to make notes that will include both the positive and the less positive aspects, and you are then able to accept the idea that every situation definitely has positive sides to it as well.

In conclusion, as I have mentioned, stress can serve as a factor of growth in our lives as long as we have learned to apply appropriate patterns of action. If we teach our brains through practice to classify stressful situations as positive, we can create a new thinking pattern for ourselves. Brain structure and function are constantly changing in response to environmental influences, so recognizing our brain's ability to change is essential.

APPENDIX

KNOW YOURSELF – HOW STRESSED ARE YOU?

The following questionnaire can illustrate the degree of stress we are in. It is important to point out that this type of questionnaire can lead to misleading results. On one hand it can be an effective diagnostic tool, and on the other it is subject to bias.

Suppose we fill out the questionnaire after a heated quarrel with our spouse. In such a situation, it is clear that the results of the questionnaire will be unduly influenced by our emotional state.

The importance of the questionnaire, however, is in raising our awareness of stress and its role in our lives. To treat stress effectively, it is advisable to have an orderly and professional diagnosis with a specialist in the field. Stress, even if it is chronic, can be treated successfully with relatively simple means. It is definitely possible to greatly reduce the effects of stress on our daily functioning and quality of life.

I have chosen to present you with a questionnaire that can give you a proper snapshot of each individual's level of stress.

There are twenty-five questions. For each question, check the value that best represents your feeling:

0 = never, 1 = rarely, 2 = sometimes, 3 = often, 4 = usually.

In the past month, to what extent have you felt:

No.	Question	Scale
1	I don't have enough time to complete all the tasks I have undertaken	01234
2	The number problems I am facing is greater than my ability to cope	01234
3	I do the work of others in addition to mine	01234
4	I have too many work / family commitments	01234
5	My confidence level is lower than I want it to be	01234
6	I have guilty feelings when I rest or do something just for myself	01234
7	I keep thinking about problems even during periods of rest	01234
8	I feel tired and worn out even after a long night's sleep	01234
9	My appetite has changed radically. I'm either hungry all the time or I have no appetite at all	01234
10	I want to win at all costs	01234
11	I have mood swings	01234
12	I want everything to be perfect in my life	01234
13	I'm constantly worried	01234
14	It's hard to fall asleep, my sleep is disturbed	01234
15	I feel discomfort / pain in one of these areas: lower back, neck, or shoulders	01234
16	I often find my mind wandering and engaging in endless thoughts	01234
17	I feel an accelerated heartbeat or spasms	01234
18	I smoke or am drinking more alcohol	01234
19	I have less leisure time to engage in hobbies and topics that interest me	01234

20	I feel nervous and frustrated by issues related to my workplace	01234
21	I feel that my life is stuck and not going anywhere	01234
22	My self-esteem is lower than I want it to be	01234
23	My expectations of those around me at home and at work are high and I am constantly disappointed by others	01234
24	The frequency of my headaches has increased	01234
25	I have little desire to go out and have fun	01234

Key to the numerical totals of the questionnaire:

- Results in the 25-50 range: It is likely that the degree of stress you are experiencing is relatively low and your probability of suffering from stress symptoms is minimal.
- 51-75 range: You are experiencing a feeling of stress, but at this stage these feelings do not have much effect on your functioning or on your quality of life. Please re-read through this book to preserve this low-level stress. If you wish, you are welcome to seek consultation from a psychotherapist, psychologist, or your family doctor.
- 76-100 range: You are experiencing a high degree of stress, a major component of which derives from personality traits, such as a feeling of not being sufficiently appreciated and low self-esteem as well as a tendency to strive for perfection. Please delve once again into the book and consult your GP for professional help.

Some tips:

First, no matter what grade or level of approval you receive, don't be stressed. Everything has a solution. Second, adopt the following guidelines:

1. Go over the questionnaire again and think if you can reduce or change one of the following measurements: level of self-confidence, self-esteem, a tendency to always seek perfection and the need to be constantly in control.

2. Start with the things you perceive as easier to modify.

3. Don't set extremely high goals and don't expect far-reaching changes to take place quickly. This is an ongoing process. Change comes in stages. Daily practice is needed for results.

4. Make sure to gain the support of friends and family. Share your feelings with those who are close to you and don't be shy about expressing yourself. You will be surprised to learn that many other people feel as you do and they are also dealing with stress of their own. Sharing will make the process easier and smoother.

5. Remember, professional help is always important and always available. Your family doctor is a good place to start!

List of References

1.   Harari, Y.N., *21 Lessons for the 21st Century.* 2018. Random House.

2.   Marsh, N., *Fat, Forty and Fired.* 2011. Random House Australia.

3.   Ursin, H. and H.R. Eriksen, *The cognitive activation theory of stress.* Psycho neuroendocrinology. 2004. 29(5): p. 567-592.

4.   *Doidge, N., The brain that changes itself: Stories of personal triumph from the frontiers of brain science. 2007. Penguin.*

5.   *Restak, R., The Naked Brain: How the Emerging Neurosociety is Changing How We Live, Work, and Love. 2006. Random House, Inc.*

6.   *Michael, E.B., et al., fMRI investigation of sentence comprehension by eye and by ear: Modality fingerprints on cognitive processes. Human brain mapping. 2001. 13(4): p. 239-252.*

7.   *Lieberman, M.D., et al., Subjective Responses to Emotional Stimuli During Labeling, Reappraisal, and Distraction. Emotion (Washington, D.C.). 2011. 11(3): p. 468-480.*

8.   *Tabibnia, G., M.D. Lieberman, and M.G. Craske, The Lasting Effect of Words on Feelings: Words May Facilitate Exposure Effects to Threatening Images.* Emotion (Washington, D.C.). 2008. 8(3): p. 307-317.

9.   *Seligman, M.E., Helplessness: On depression, development, and death. 1975.*

10.   *Sarno, J.E., The divided mind: The epidemic of mind body disorders. 2009. Harper Collins.*

11.   Frances, A., *The new crisis of confidence in psychiatric diagnosis.* Annals of internal medicine. 2013. 159(3): p. 221-222.

12. Robertson, I., *The Stress Test: How Pressure Can Make You Stronger and Sharper. 2016. Bloomsbury Publishing.*

13. Yerkes, R.M. and J.D. Dodson, *The relation of strength of stimulus to rapidity of habit — formation.* Journal of comparative neurology and psychology. 1908. 18(5): p. 459-482.

14. Stossel,S., *My Age of Anxiety*, Vintage, 2014.

15. Collins, J. and M.T. Hansen, *Great by Choice: Uncertainty, Chaos and Luck-Why some thrive despite them all. 2011. Random House.*

16. Ein-Dor, T., M. Mikulincer, and P.R. Shaver, *Effective Reaction to Danger Attachment Insecurities Predict Behavioral Reactions to an Experimentally Induced Threat Above and Beyond General Personality Traits. Social Psychological and Personality Science.* 2011. 2(5): p. 467-473.

17. Chapman, J., *Anxiety and defective decision making: an elaboration of the group think model. Management Decision.* 2006. 44(10): p. 1391-1404.

18. Penney, A.M., VC. Miedema, and D. Mazmanian, *Intelligence and emotional disorders: Is the worrying and ruminating mind a more intelligent mind? Personality and Individual Differences.* 2015. 74: p. 90-93.

19. Treynor, W., R. Gonzalez, and S. Nolen-Hoeksema, *Rumination reconsidered: A psychometric analysis.* Cognitive therapy and research. 2003. 27(3): p. 247-259.

20. Richardsen, A.M. and S.B. Matthiesen, *Managers: Less stress when work relationships are good, in ScienceDaily. 2014.*

21. Grove, A.S., *Only the paranoid survive: How to exploit the crisis points that challenge every company and career. 1996. Broadway Business.*

22. Sweller, J., *Cognitive load during problem solving: Effects on*

learning. Cognitive science. 1988. 12(2): p. 257-285.

23. *Lazarus, R.S. and S. Folkman, Stress, appraisal, and coping. 1984. New York: Springer.*

24. *Folkman, S., Stress: appraisal and coping, in Encyclopedia of behavioral medicine. 2013. Springer. p. 1913-1915.*

25. Ben-Avi, N., S. Toker, and D. Heller, *"If stress is good for me, it's probably good for you too:" Stress mindset and judgment of others 'strain.* Journal of Experimental Social Psychology. 2018. 74: p. 98-110.

26. Bortner, R. and R. Rosenman, *The measurement of pattern A behavior.* Journal of chronic diseases. 1967. 20(7): p. 525.

27. Costa, P.T. and R.R. McCrae, *The NEO personality inventory,* 1985.

28. McCrae, R.R. and PT. Costa Jr, *Personality trait structure as a human universal.* American psychologist. 1997. 52(5): p. 509.

29. *Meyer Stamp, E., The Relationships between Perceived Stress, The Big Five Inventory, The Five-Facet Mindfulness Questionnaire, and Yoga. 2016.*

30. McCrae, R.R. and P.T. Costa Jr, *A five-factor theory of personality. Handbook of personality: Theory and research.* Vol. 2. 1999. p. 139-153.

31. *Hankin, B.L., Personality and depressive symptoms: Stress generation and cognitive vulnerabilities to depression in a prospective daily diary study. Journal of Social and Clinical Psychology, 29(4): p. 369-401.*

32. *Esia-Donkoh, K., D. Yelkpieri, and K. Esia-Donkoh, Coping with Stress: Strategies Adopted by Students at the Winneba Campus of University of Education, Winneba, Ghana. Online Submission. 2011.*

33. Morgan, C.A.I., et al., *Relationship among Plasma Cortisol, Catecholamines, Neuropeptide Y and Human Performance during Exposure to Uncontrollable Stress. Psychosomatic Medicine.* 2001. 63(3): p. 412-422.

34. Kagan, J., *Temperament and the Reactions to Unfamiliarity. Child Development.* 1997. 68(1): p. 139-143.

35. Richardson, K.M. and H.R. Rothstein, *Effects of occupational stress management intervention programs: a meta-analysis. Journal of occupational health psychology.* 2008. 13(1): p. 69.

36. Witkowski, T., *Thirty-five years of research on Neuro-Linguistic Programming. NLP research data base. State of the art or pseudoscientific decoration? Polish Psychological Bulletin.* 2010. 41(2): p. 58-66.

37. Moss, D., *Biofeedback, mind-body medicine, and the higher limits of human nature. Humanistic and transpersonal psychology: A historical and biographical sourcebook.* 1999. p. 145-161.

38. Kabat-Zinn, J., *Mindfulness — based interventions in context: past, present, and future. Clinical psychology: Science and practice.* 2003. 10(2): p. 144-156.

39. Kabat-Zinn, J., et al., *Effectiveness of a meditation-based stress reduction program in the treatment of anxiety disorders.* 1992.

40. Grossman, P., et al., *Mindfulness-based stress reduction and health benefits: A meta-analysis.* Journal of psychosomatic research. 2004. 57(1): p. 35-43.

41. Strauss, C., et al., *Mindfulness-Based Interventions for People Diagnosed with a Current Episode of an Anxiety or Depressive Disorder: A Meta-Analysis of Randomised Controlled Trials.* 2014.

42. Holzel, B.K., et al., *How does mindfulness meditation work? Proposing mechanisms of action from a conceptual and neural*

perspective. Perspectives on psychological science. 2011. 6(6): p. 537-559.

43. Holzel, B.K., et al., *Mindfulness practice leads to increases in regional brain gray matter density.* Psychiatry Research: Neuroimaging. 2011. 191(1): p. 36-43.

44. *Chiesa, A. and A. Serretti, Mindfulness-Based Stress Reduction for Stress Management in Healthy People: A Review and Meta-Analysis. The Journal of Alternative and Complementary Medicine. 2009. 15(5): p. 593-600.*

45. *Emmons, R.A. and M.E. McCullough, Counting blessings versus burdens: an experimental investigation of gratitude and subjective well-being in daily life. Journal of personality and social psychology. 2003. 84(2): p. 377.*

46. *Puterman, E., et al., Determinants of telomere attrition over one year in healthy older women: Stress and health behaviors matter. Psychiatry. 2015. 20(4): p. 529-535.*

47. *O'Donovan, A., et al., Pessimism correlates with leukocyte telomere shortness and elevated interleukin-6 in post-menopausal women. Brain, behavior, and immunity. 2009. 23(4): p. 446-449.*

48. *Ikeda, A., et al., Pessimistic orientation in relation to telomere length in older men: the VA Normative Aging Study. Psychoneurosis endocrinology. 2014. 42: p. 68-76.*

49. Wegner, D.M., *When the antidote is the poison: Ironic mental control processes.* Psychological Science. 1997. 8(3): p. 148-150.

50. *Wegner, D.M., How to Think, Say, or Do Precisely the Worst Thing for Any Occasion. Science. 2009.*

51. Poe, E.A., Graham's Lady's and Gentleman's Magazine, 1845.

52. Zainuddin, M.S.A. and S. Thuret, *Nutrition, adult hippocampal neurogenesis and mental health.* British medical bulletin. 2012. p. lds021.

53. Kramer, A.F., et al., *Ageing, fitness and neurocognitive function*. Nature. 1999. 400(6743): p. 418.

54. Winter, B., et al., *High impact running improves learning*. Neurobiology of learning and memory. 2007. 87(4): p. 597-609.

55. Ploughman, M., *Exercise is brain food: The effects of physical activity on cognitive function*. Developmental Neurorehabilitation. 2008. 11(3): p. 236-240.

56. *Vancampfort, D., et al., Effects of progressive muscle relaxation on state anxiety and subjective well-being in people with schizophrenia: a randomized controlled trial. Clinical Rehabilitation. 2011. 25(6): p. 567-575.*

57. Carney, D.R., A.J. Cuddy, and A.J. Yap, *Power posing: Brief nonverbal displays affect neuroendocrine levels and risk tolerance*. Psychological science. 2010. 21(10): p. 1363-1368.

58. *Shafir, T., et al., Emotion regulation through execution, observation, and imagery of emotional movements. 2013.*

59. Seelig, T., *inGenius: A Crash Course on Creativity*. 2012. New York: HarperCollins.

60. *Wedell-Wedellsborg, T., Are You Solving the Right Problems? Harvard Business Review. 2017.*

61. *Robertson, I., What simple actions lift mood? 2016.*

62. Jarratt, D. and S. Gammon, *'We had the most wonderful times': seaside nostalgia at a British resort*. Tourism Recreation Research. 2016. 41(2): p. 123-133.

63. Ibid.

64. *Cheung, W.-Y., et al., Back to the future: Nostalgia increases optimism*. Personality and Social Psychology Bulletin. 2013. 39(11): p. 1484-1496.

65. Routledge, C., et al., *Nostalgia as a resource for psychological health and well — being*. Social and Personality Psychology

Compass. 2013. 7(11): p. 808-818.

66. Sedikides, C., et al., *Nostalgia: Past, present, and future.* Current Directions in Psychological Science. 2008. 17(5): p. 304-307.

67. *Frankl, V.E., Man's Search for Meaning: An Introduction to Logotherapy: a Newly Revised and Enlarged Edition of from Death-camp to Existentialism. 1962. Beacon Press.*

68. Mani, M., et al., *Review and evaluation of mindfulness-based iPhone apps.* JMIR mHealth and uHealth. 2015. 3(3).

69. *Lyubomisrsky, S., The how of happiness: A new approach to getting the life you want. 2007. New York. The Penguin Press.*

70. Gilbert, D., *Stumbling on happiness.* 2009. Vintage Canada.

71. *Achor, S., The happiness advantage: The seven principles of positive psychology that fuel success and performance at work. 2011. Random House.*

72. *Graham, L., Bouncing Back: Rewiring Your Brain for Maximum Resilience and Well-Being. 2013.*

73. *PwC, Creating a mentally healthy workplace. Return on investment analysis. 2014.*

74. 74. Varghese, L. and L.K. Barber, *Are Your Employees Prone to Workplace Stress? Mentoring May Help.* APA Center for Organizational Excellence: Good Company Newsletter. 2014. 8(9).

75. Kubesch, S., et al., *Aerobic endurance exercise improves executive functions in depressed patients.* Journal of Clinical Psychiatry. 2003. 64(9): p. 1005-1012.

76. *Ratey, J.J. and E. Hagerman, Spark: The revolutionary new science of exercise and the brain. 2008. Little Brown & Company.*

77. Mednick, S. and M. Ehrman, *Take a Nap! Change Your Life.* 2006. New York. Workman Publishing Company.

78. Adam, T.C. and E.S. Epel, *Stress, eating and the reward system.* Physiology & behavior. 2007. 91(4): p. 449-458.

79. Amichai,Y. Shaat Hesed (An Hour of Grace), Schocken, 1986

80. Bonanno, G.A., et al., *Resilience to Loss and Chronic Grief: A Prospective Study from Preloss to 18-Months Postloss.* Journal of Personality and Social Psychology. 2002. 83(5): p. 1150-1164.

81. Burnett, D., *Idiot Brain: What Your Head is Really Up to.* 2016. WW Norton & Company.

82. *Lipton, B.H., The Biology of Belief 10th Anniversary Edition. Unleashing the Power of Consciousness, Matter & Miracles.* 2015. Hay House, Inc.